Paediatrics and Medications

A Resource for Guiding Nurses in Paediatric Medication Administration

T0289441

Paediatrics and Medications

A Resource for Guiding Nurses in Paediatric Medication Administration

Kerry Reid-Searl (AM)

PhD, Mclin Ed, BHlth Sc, RN, RM
Professor of Simulation and Innovation at the University of Tasmania
Emeritus Professor at CQUniversity
Adjunct Professor at Monash University, Australia

Pauline Davies

BHlth Sc Nursing, Grad Dip, RN
Current practising clinician and Nurse Unit Manager
Central Queensland Hospital and Health Service
Queensland, Australia

Rinnah Peacock

BHlth Sc Nursing, Grad Cert, RN
Current practising clinician and Nurse Educator
Central Queensland Hospital and Health Service
Queensland, Australia

ELSEVIER

ELSEVIER

ISBN: 978-0-7295-4464-1

Notice

This publication has been carefully reviewed and checked to ensure that the content is as accurate and current as possible at time of publication. We would recommend, however, that the reader verify any procedures, treatments, drug dosages or legal content described in this book. Neither the author, the contributors, nor the publisher assume any liability for injury and/or damage to persons or property arising from any error in or omission from this publication.

National Library of Australia Cataloguing-in-Publication Data

---

A catalogue record for this book is available from the National Library of Australia

NATIONAL LIBRARY OF AUSTRALIA

Content Strategist: Natalie Hunt
Content Project Manager: Fariha Nadeem
Edited by Lynn Watt
Proofread by Annabel Adair
Copyrights Coordinator: Ashwini Dhayalan
Cover Designer: Gopalakrishnan Venkatraman
Index by Innodata

Typeset by GW Tech

Printed in China by 1010 Printing International Ltd

Last digit is the print number: 9 8 7 6 5 4 3 2 1

Dedicated to all the passionate paediatric nurses we have had the pleasure of working with.

About the book

This guide has been prepared with an emphasis on the process of medication administration to the paediatric patient. It is not a resource relating to specific medications or pharmacology.

While this guide may be a useful resource it does not replace or override guidelines, policy and procedures of the organisation in which an individual using this guide is employed.

While every effort has been made to ensure that the content of this guide is accurate, no responsibility will be taken for inaccuracies, omissions or errors. The authors do not accept liability to any person or information obtained from this publication or for loss or damages incurred because of the reliance on the material contained in this guide.

Introduction

Paediatrics and medications: a resource for guiding nurses in paediatric medication administration is a guide only. Nurses have a significant responsibility in safely administering medication to the paediatric patient. This resource is meant to be a companion guide to pharmacology texts by providing complementary information about the process of medication administration to children with an emphasis on medication safety.

The paediatric patient receiving medication

The aim of administering medication to the paediatric patient is to do so in a safe and efficient manner. The nurse needs to understand:

- Their own scope of practice
- Basic maths and calculating drug dosages
- Assessment of the paediatric patient
- Consent
- The education of the paediatric patient and caregiver about medications
- Legal requirements and responsibilities associated with medication administration to the paediatric patient
- Administration considerations for the paediatric patient.

Contents

Contributor List

Shandell Elmer RN BA (Hons) PhD

Associate Professor
Course Coordinator Bachelor of Nursing with Honours
School of Nursing
College of Health and Medicine
Newnham Campus, University of Tasmania
Tasmania

Reviewer List

Darlene Archer RN
Lecturer in Nursing
City East Campus
University of South Australia
South Australia

Andrea Chelkowski RN, B Prof Honours Paed, Grad Cert, Grad Dip Paed
Associate Unit Nurse Manager, Royal Hobart Hospital, Tasmanian Health Service
Registered Nurse, Aged Care Uniting Agewell, Sorell, Tasmania
Registered Nurse, Southern Cross Care
Agency Registered Nurse, Redstone Recruitment
Tasmania

Emma Collins RN, MN, PhD Candidate
Senior Professional Practice Child Health
University of Otago, Dunedin campus
New Zealand

Julie Ferguson RN, Grad Dip HSM, Mas Nurs (Advanced pract), Ma Nurs (Nurse pract), Grad cert LTHE
Lecturer in Nursing/Mental Health
Charles Sturt University
Bathurst, Wagga Wagga

Elyce Kenny RN BN, Grad Cert (Nurs Ed), Grad Dip Paed Child & Yth Health Nursing
Lecturer and Course Coordinator, University of Adelaide-Adelaide Nursing School
Registered Nurse-Women's and Children's Hospital
South Australia

Andrea Middleton RN, MN (Paeds)

Lecturer
School of Nursing
College of Health and Medicine
University of Tasmania, Hobart, Tasmania

Sarah Stenson B Nurs, M Nurs

Lecturer in Nursing
Charles Sturt University
Bathurst, Wagga Wagga

Debra Surman RN BN MN Grad Cert Emergency Nsg

Lecturer
College of Nursing and Health Sciences
Flinders University, Adelaide
South Australia

Scope of practice, maths and calculating drug dosages

Kerry Reid-Searl, Pauline Davies, Rinnah Peacock

Scope of practice

Nurses need to ascertain whether administering medication to a paediatric patient is within their scope of practice. The table below provides an overview of the scope of practice for different nursing roles in the Australian context.

Bachelor Degree Nursing Students or Diploma Nursing Students	Yes	If content has been covered in the relevant university or diploma course, assessment has occurred, it is within the stated scope of practice and direct supervision is present. However, students should always confirm their scope of practice with their program coordinator. A student cannot be a second independent person checking medication
Assistant in Nursing (AIN)	No	This is not in the AIN's scope of practice

| Graduate Diploma/ Enrolled Nurse (EN) | Yes | The EN must have medication endorsement and a second approved person checking the medication |
| Graduate/Registered Nurse (RN) | Yes | The RN must follow organisation policy regarding checking the medication |

Basic maths and calculating drug dosages

There is a basic level of maths that nurses should be well versed in with regards to safe medication administration. The following section addresses some important elements (Tables 1.1–1.6).

Basic formulae for calculation of drug doses

ORAL MEDICATIONS SOLIDS/LIQUIDS

$$\frac{\text{Strength required}}{\text{Strength in stock}} \times \frac{\text{Volume}}{1} = \text{Amount required}$$

TABLE 1.1 24-hour clock		
	AM	PM
12	1200	2400
1	0100	1300
2	0200	1400
3	0300	1500
4	0400	1600
5	0500	1700
6	0600	1800
7	0700	1900
8	0800	2000
9	0900	2100
10	1000	2200
11	1100	2300
12	1200	2400

Box 1.1
An example of dose calculation by weight and recommended dosage

Step 1

Look up in the relevant resource, for example, the *Australian Medicines Handbook* (AMH), MIMS online or Hospital IV Guidelines for the recommended dosage of a prescribed drug per kg
For example:
A paediatric patient is to be given ampicillin. The recommended dosage is 80 mg/kg/day divided by four doses over four doses over 24 hours (per day). The nurse must check the single dose prescribed
The paediatric patient weight is 27 kg:
* *27 kg × 80 mg/kg/day = 2160 mg/day*
Then:
* *2160 mg ÷ 4 doses = 540 mg/dose*
Check that the dose prescribed is within the recommended range. If not, do not proceed until the dose is questioned with the prescribing doctor

Step 2

If the dose is within the recommended range, use the appropriate formula to work out how much to give
If the doctor has prescribed a dose of 540 mg and the label on the ampicillin bottle reads 100 mg of ampicillin in every 5 mL, the nurse uses the following formula to work out the amount to give:

$$\frac{\textbf{Strenght required}}{\textbf{Stored Strength}} \times \frac{\textbf{Volume}}{\textbf{1}}$$

$$\frac{540\,\text{mg}}{100} \times \frac{5}{1} = 5.4 \text{ mL}$$

Step 3

The workings of the calculations should be double-checked with a second medication-endorsed person

TABLE 1.2 Example of fraction, decimal and percentage conversion

FRACTION	SIMPLIFIED FRACTION	TERMINOLOGY	DECIMAL FRACTION	PERCENTAGE
10/100	1/10	One-tenth	0.1	10%
25/100	1/4	One-quarter	0.25	25%
33/100	1/3	One-third	0.33	33%
50/100	1/2	One-half	0.5	50%

TABLE 1.3 Abbreviation and meaning

ABBREVIATION	MEANING
mL	millilitre
L	litre
kg	kilogram
g	gram
mg	milligram
mcg or microg	microgram
Unit(s)	International Units
m	metre
cm	centimetre

TABLE 1.4 Metric equivalents

VOLUME	
1 litre (L)	1000 millilitres (mL)
MASS	
1 kilogram (kg)	1000 grams (g)
1 gram (g)	1000 milligrams (mg)
1 milligram (mg)	1000 micrograms (microg)
LENGTH	
1 kilometre (km)	1000 metres (m)
1 metre (m)	100 centimetres (cm)
1 centimetre (cm)	10 millimetres (mm)

TABLE 1.5 Example of equivalents

0.5 kilograms	500 grams
0.5 grams	500 milligrams
0.5 milligrams	500 micrograms
0.5 litres	500 millilitres

TABLE 1.6 Common intravenous fluids selected for paediatrics	
Sodium chloride 0.9%	Isotonic
Sodium chloride 0.9% and glucose 5%	Hypertonic
Glucose 5% in water	Isotonic

Tablet example: You are required to give paracetamol 1000 mg to a 17-year-old who weighs 80 kg. The stock available is 500 mg tablets.
The calculation is as follows:

$$\frac{1000 \text{ mg}}{500 \text{ mg}} \times \frac{1}{1} = 2 \text{ tablets}$$

Mixture example: You are required to give a 4-year-old paediatric patient who weighs 15 kg, paracetamol 225 mg. The stock strength available in elixir form is paracetamol 100 mg per mL.
The calculation is as follows:

$$\frac{225 \text{ mg}}{100 \text{ mg}} \times \frac{1}{1} = 2.25 \text{ mL}$$

PARENTAL MEDICATION

Solutions (IM, IV injections)
The formula is:

$$\frac{\text{Strength required}}{\text{Strength in stock}} \times \frac{\text{Volume of stock strength}}{1} = \text{Volume required}$$

Example: You are required to give a 15-year-old who weighs 65 kg, morphine 5 mg IMI (intramuscular injection). The stock strength available are morphine ampoules 10 mg per mL.
The calculation is as follows:

$$\frac{5 \text{ mg}}{10 \text{ mg}} \times \frac{1}{1} = 0.5 \text{ mL}$$

POWDERS
It is essential that the manufacturer's directions are followed. The directions will indicate the dilution and then the formulae can be applied.

Intravenous fluids infusions

When intravenous (IV) solutions are administered to the paediatric patient, an infusion pump and burette should be used. The volume in the burette should be set, for example, per hour. At each hour the volume infused should be checked and recorded on a fluid balance chart. Additionally, when intravenous fluids are infusing, the infusion site should be checked for stability and for signs of complications such as phlebitis or infiltration.

The volume of intravenous fluids to be ordered by the medical officer and administered to the paediatric patient is determined by the weight, age and hydration status of the child. The nurse has a responsibility to know what the volume of fluid per hour the paediatric patient should have.

Full maintenance of IV fluid rates can be calculated using Table 1.7.

TABLE 1.7   Maintenance intravenous fluids per hour

WEIGHT (KG)	ML/HOUR
3–10 kg	4 × weight
10–20 kg	40 plus 2 × (weight minus 10)
20–60 kg	60 plus 1 × (weight minus 20)
Greater than 60	100 mL/hour

Example of calculated intravenous (IV) fluids per hour.

Please be reminded that it is the medical officer who orders the fluid and determines the rate; however, the nurse has a responsibility to understand what is considered to be an appropriate volume of fluid per hour according to, among other factors, the patient's hydration status, weight and age.

A paediatric patient weighs 10 kg.
The formula for the 10-kg patient is:
4 × weight (10 kg) = 40 mL per hour.
A paediatric patient weighs 20 kg.

The formula for the 20-kg patient is:
40 + 2 × (20–10) = 60 mL per hour.

When an IV fluid volume is ordered by the medical officer, including the set timeframe to be delivered overwritten on a fluid order chart, the nurse can then work out the volume per hour.

Example: You are caring for a 15-year-old who weighs 65 kg (maintenance fluid is 100 mL per hour). The fluid order is for 1 L of 0.9% sodium chloride over 12 hours. To work out volume per hour, the calculation is as follows:
Volume of fluid divided by time in hours = Volume per hour.

Example: 1000 mL of 0.9 % saline over 12 hours:
1000 divided by 12 = 83 mL per hour.

Assessment of the paediatric patient, consent and legal considerations

Rinnah Peacock, Kerry Reid-Searl, Pauline Davies

Assessment

The assessment of the paediatric patient should be holistic and include the paediatric patient's developmental stage, their psychosocial situation, medical conditions, reasons for medication, relevant history, a physical assessment, other medications currently being taken, allergies and weight (Tiziani 2017). It is not within the scope of this guide to consider all elements of assessment; however, it is important to note the importance of age and weight.

AGE AND WEIGHT VARIATIONS

Medication doses for paediatric patients are usually based on the paediatric patient's age, weight and/or body surface area. Therefore, an accurate weight on admission is required for all paediatric patients.

The paediatric patient average weight is used for some medications to ensure an effective medication dose is administered.

The average weight is used particularly if a paediatric patient is significantly overweight or underweight for their age. In addition to the assessment of the child for medication administration, the six rights of medication administration must be adhered to, as discussed further in Chapter 4.

Table 2.1 portrays the average weight according to age.

TABLE 2.1 Average weight according to age		
AGE	WEIGHT (KG)	HEIGHT (CM)
Birth (at term)	3.3	50
1 month	4.4	55
2 months	5.4	58
3 months	6.1	61
4 months	6.7	63
6 months	7.6	67
1 year	9	75
2 years	12	87
3 years	14	96
4 years	16	103
5 years	18	110
6 years	21	115
8 years	25	127
10 years	33	139
12 years	41	150
14-year-old boy	51	164
14-year-old girl	50	160

(AMH Australian Children's Dosing Companion 2022.)

Consent

As with any procedure a nurse performs, consent is important and required when administering medications. Informed consent is the process between patient and nurse where information is communicated back and forth to ensure understanding (Clinical Excellence Queensland 2023). This is an important aspect of providing holistic, patient-centred care. For paediatric patients this consent is often given by the parents, but it is prudent to still involve the paediatric patient in the process. Involving the paediatric patient in this consent process will most often yield a positive procedural process for which consent is sought.

Gillick Competency is used throughout Australia in relation to capacity to consent. Please check your state health guides for all other aspects relating to consent, as they may differ from state to state.

When gaining consent for a paediatric patient, some situations need considering:

1. **Is the paediatric patient able to provide consent?**

   YES

Then all elements of valid consent must be adhered to. The nurse should pay particular attention to:

- Checking that the consent is informed.
  - Has the paediatric patient been provided with information needed to make an informed decision?
- Does the paediatric patient have the capacity to understand the information and consequences of the decision?
  - Refer to Gillick Competency.
- Is the paediatric patient providing the consent voluntarily?
  - Not being pressured by caregivers/friends or any other influence.

(Hockenberry, Wilson & Rogers 2019.)

If the paediatric patient is not able to consent, then the caregiver should provide consent with the nurse adhering to all the above elements. The parents must also have capacity to provide consent.

- Make sure they are understanding what they are consenting to
  - For example, English may not be the parents' first language.
- Are they mentally fit to provide consent?
  - For example, not suffering from postnatal depression.

   NO

- Is the paediatric patient of the legal age to provide consent?
  - This is different for each state in Australia; please refer to your local state health policy and procedures.
- Is the paediatric patient under the guardianship of the state?
  - This requires the nurse to refer to the *Child Protection Act 1999* (legislation.qld.gov.au).

Each paediatric patient under the guardianship of the state may fall under a different carer agreement and the authorities must be contacted to see who is able to give consent for medical examinations/treatment. The carer agreements are always changing (a living document) and need to be reviewed to ensure the right authorities have been contacted for consent.

2. **Is the paediatric patient under the *Mental Health Act*?**

If a paediatric patient is under the *Mental Health Act 2016* (Queensland Government 2023), nurses need to find the legislation relevant to their jurisdiction. If the patient is not able to consent to treatment due to their mental illness, an authorised doctor may make a treatment order. The doctor must be satisfied that the treatment criteria apply and that there is no less restrictive way of providing treatment and care for the person.

Mental Health Acts (MHAs) enable the involuntary commitment and treatment of people suffering acute psychiatric illness. Each jurisdiction in Australia and New Zealand has its own MHA and attempts to balance civil liberties with the need to prevent serious harm and provide care (The Royal Australian and New Zealand College of Psychiatrists 2023).

Legal considerations

Before a drug can be administered safely, the nurse must know the legal aspects of drug administration and specific considerations for the paediatric patient. This includes:

- Knowledge in laws governing the possession, use and dispensation of medication; and
- The directives of the nurse's registering body on the administration of medications to the paediatric patient.

Nurses also need to understand the requirements of the employing organisation in terms of occupational health and safety, which relate to the safe storage, handling and use of medications. It is important to be familiar with policy around the latter. The legal aspects for safe medication administration are addressed further in Chapter 5.

Educational preparation of the paediatric patient and caregiver for medication administration

Shandell Elmer

Administering medications to the paediatric patient requires careful consideration of all the factors that impact on the paediatric patient's ability to understand the information provided about the medication and follow the directions given. As part of family and patient-centred care, support also needs to be given to the paediatric patient's caregiver to ensure they understand their paediatric patient's medications and are equipped to safely manage these ongoing if required. Preparing the paediatric patient for medication administration requires consideration of the health literacy development needs of the paediatric patient and the health literacy of their caregiver.

Health literacy is the ability of people to access health information and services. Health literacy skills are more than the individual's literacy and numeracy. People use their health literacy skills to navigate the health system, find and appraise health information, ask questions from their healthcare provider, manage their own health, and draw on their social networks to support their health. Health literacy is a social determinant of health and is the result of the complex interplay with other social determinants. For example, level of educational attainment can influence someone's health literacy. In order to improve nurse–patient communication the health literacy strengths, needs and preferences of the patient must be considered, and just as importantly, it requires the nurse to be health literacy responsive. A health literacy responsive nurse will recognise and accommodate these strengths, needs and preferences to create an enabling environment to optimise the patient's access to and engagement with health information and services (Australian Institute of Health and Welfare 2022; Osborne et al 2022).

The process for effective patient education is based on these four components:

- Assessment
- Planning
- Implementation; and
- Evaluation (Bastable 2016).

Assessment

Consider the paediatric patient's and their caregiver's:

- Prior education about medications
- Readiness to learn
- Culture and preferred language
- Preferred learning styles
- Literacy levels
- Paediatric patient's stage of development

Assessing the paediatric patient and their caregiver

THE PAEDIATRIC PATIENT AND CAREGIVER'S READINESS TO LEARN

The paediatric patient and their caregiver's ability to engage in medication education is impacted by physical, emotional and mental wellbeing.

The PEEK model (Kitchie 2006) to assess readiness to learn can guide a holistic nursing assessment:

- Physical readiness
- Emotional readiness
- Experiential readiness
- Knowledge readiness.

Communication aids may be needed to augment or provide alternative to speech:

- Reading glasses
- Hearing aids
- Communication devices
- Boards
- Cards.

Pain or discomfort, anxiety, stress or fear, will all impact on the paediatric patient and their caregiver's ability to receive and understand health information, and need to be prioritised. The nurse needs to ensure the paediatric patient and their caregiver are as comfortable as possible and monitor their status throughout the education session.

The timing of the education session needs to be matched with the paediatric patient and their caregiver's readiness to learn. Finding 'teachable moments' when opportunities arise as part of other aspects of nursing care can be helpful for reinforcing information and checking understanding. Informing the paediatric patient and their caregiver ahead of time that the nurse wants to spend some time discussing medication will help them to prepare (e.g., to prepare their questions and know what to expect).

CULTURE AND PREFERRED LANGUAGE OF THE PAEDIATRIC PATIENT AND THEIR CAREGIVER

The nurse needs to assess whether there are any language barriers and/or cultural disparities that may impact on the paediatric patient and their caregiver's ability to engage with medication education. The nurse should ensure that the medication education is delivered in culturally safe and sensitive ways. The nurse also needs to be aware of any cultural values that may influence beliefs and behaviours around medication and the nurse–patient/caregiver interaction. These considerations include:

- Non-verbal communication and body language
- Parental involvement in giving medication

- Family belief system around medication
- Direct and non-judgemental questioning.

English-language proficiency will also play a significant role in the ability of the paediatric patient and their caregiver to engage with medication education. Using interpreters can help to overcome language barriers. However, some difficulties may remain as the interpreter will convey the information using the same medical terms used by the nurse, which may not be readily understood or translated into other languages. If translated materials are used, these need to be easily understood and be free of jargon and complex medical terms.

LITERACY AND NUMERACY

The literacy and numeracy ability of the paediatric patient and their caregiver will determine the format and content of the delivery of the medication information. This includes their proficiency in English, as well as in other languages, which is also an important consideration for the translation of written materials as people may not be literate in their preferred language. Medication management for children requires numeracy skills, for example, calculating medication dose based on body weight, measuring medication, timing of medication doses. The nurse should consider the inclusion of easy to administer (verbally as well as written), simple and short screening measures for literacy and numeracy that can be used in a non-shaming and non-judgemental way, for example, *The Newest Vital Sign* (The Newest Vital Sign 2023).

Information should be developmentally appropriate for the paediatric patient and be clearly understood by the caregiver. This may require tailoring of information and the use of a variety of teaching methods and materials.

There is an array of information on literacy and numeracy in education; however, some key points the nurse should consider are:

- Using plain language for the paediatric patient and/or caregiver – avoid medical language, terminology and abbreviations, which may be confusing
- Ensure that written information, such as a pamphlet, is easily understood
- Choosing a mode of delivery that is preferred by the paediatric patient and their caregiver and matches with their learning styles

- Using strategies to lessen the need for numeracy, for example, pre-packaged/dispensing aids for medications, medications formulated in the required doses, photos of the number of tablets or amount of medication required
- Reducing the literacy and numeracy burden.

These audio-visual resources demonstrate the importance of being patient-focused when developing materials by highlighting the ways that healthcare providers can become so ingrained in their own ways of communicating with each other, using jargon and complex language, for example, that they are unaware of how difficult it is for others (patients) to understand.

Planning the education

PLANNING THE NURSE–PATIENT/CAREGIVER INTERACTION

The nurse needs to identify the learning needs of the paediatric patient and their caregiver.

To avoid giving more information than is wanted and needed:
- Ask open-ended questions
- What do they already know?
- What do they need and want to know?
- Assess prior knowledge.
  Learning needs (Kitchie 2006) can be prioritised as:
- Mandatory (essential or critical) e.g. recognising adverse reactions
- Desirable (related to the quality use of medicines)
- Possible (nice to know).
  Planning considerations:
- Length of time – time to ask questions, take on board the information, not feel rushed
- Timing – readiness to learn
- Frequency – learning needs and preferred learning style.
  Language considerations:
- Use conversational language that is easy to understand
- Avoid clinical overtones
- Reduce anxiety and fear with less formal discussions
- Use contextually relevant examples
- Avoid metaphors and abstract concepts
- Use realistic and relevant images and teaching aides (e.g. do not use oranges to demonstrate injection technique)

- Avoid jargon and acronyms
- Explain medical terms in lay language
- Consider the developmental age of the paediatric patient.
  Plan to use educational materials:
- Consider different learning styles
- 'Part task trainers'
- Equipment
- Flow charts
- Drawings
- Anatomical models.

Remember that the paediatric patient and caregiver may need to put this information into the context of their daily lives if the medication is to be used long term. Therefore, ask questions about their daily routines in order to identify circumstances that may help to reinforce medication management, for example, meal times, bed times.

Preparing the environment

The environment needs to be conducive to learning and help the paediatric patient and their caregiver to engage with the medication education:

- Ensure the space is free from distractions and disruptions
- Avoid background noises especially intermittent noises as these are more distracting
- Check the space offers auditory and visual privacy
- Create a non-threatening setting, keeping in mind clinical spaces can be intimidating for some people
- Have all relevant educational materials ready
- If medications are long term, ensure the equipment and materials used are similar to those available in the home environment.

Implementing the key learning strategies

WAYS PEOPLE LEARN

Understanding and identifying the preferred learning style(s) is important for determining the approaches used within the nurse–patient/caregiver interaction. The paediatric patient and their caregiver may have other ways that they learn outside of their communication and interaction with the nurse. These include community conversations, the arts, printed materials, conventional mass media and digital media. Identifying the other ways that the paediatric patient and their caregiver learn will support the development and delivery of information.

LEARNING STYLES

Learners are often multimodal, that is, they learn in more than one way, but usually have a preferred way. Learning modalities include visual, auditory, reading/writing and kinaesthetic (Fleming & Mills 1992). In delivering education, understanding the paediatric patient and their caregiver's learning style is important. Table 3.1 reflects different learning styles and strategies that may be useful to assist in education sessions. It is often useful to include more than one learning modality.

CONTENT TO BE INCLUDED IN EDUCATION

Medication education needs to cover the following points:
- Advising why the medication is required
- Actions of the medication
- Correct dose
- How it is to be administered
- Time of administration
- Side effects
- Special considerations

TABLE 3.1 Strategies for different modalities of learning	
MODALITIES FOR LEARNING INFORMATION	**STRATEGIES/EXAMPLES**
Visual – by showing	Charts, diagrams, presentations, pictures, cards, computer activities, puppets, drawing
Auditory – by listening	Vocal explanation, reading out aloud, podcasts, audio files, one-on-one conversations, oral presentations
Reading and writing	Written information on sheets, books, pamphlets, websites
Kinaesthetic – by doing	Hands-on activities, touch, role play, puppets, playdough, demonstrations, simulations

- Clarification on misconceptions that may arise – for example, antibiotic medications need to be taken until the course is completed not only until when the patient is feeling better
- What to do if the patient refuses, spits or vomits.

If a paediatric patient requires medication ongoing (after discharge), the caregiver must also know:

- How to accurately read the label on the medication, including the paediatric patient's name on the label
- What the active ingredients are
- The difference between generic and trade names of the medication
- The dose according to age and weight
- How often to administer
- If the medication needs to be given with food
- Where to find the expiry date.

These points do not need to be covered in only one session. Depending on the learning needs and preferences of the paediatric patient and their caregiver, these topics may need to be covered in multiple sessions. Prioritising the content will also help to determine the sequence of delivery.

While delivering the medication education, the nurse should invite the paediatric patient and their caregiver to make notes, draw or otherwise make a record of the information. This may include an audio recording if everyone agrees. This is important to enable the paediatric patient and their caregiver to record the information in ways that make sense to them. They may also write down their questions during the session to ask at the end or at a later session.

A useful tool to support patient engagement in the medication education process has been developed by the World Health Organization (WHO 2019). While this tool has been developed for use by adults, it may assist the paediatric patient's caregiver to manage their paediatric patient medication. The tool identifies five moments where action by the patient or caregiver can greatly reduce the risk of harm associated with medication use. These five moments are:

1. Starting a medication
2. Taking a medication
3. Adding a medication
4. Reviewing medications
5. Stopping a medication

The tool includes five questions for each of these moments to be answered by the patient with the assistance of their health-care provider.

Evaluating the teaching and learning

A collaborative communication model such as 'Ask-Tell-Ask' (assess understanding, provide clear explanations, check understanding) is a useful framework for the nurse–patient/caregiver interaction. Checking understanding is key to evaluating the effectiveness of the medication education (Badaczewski et al 2017).

Chunk and check:

- Break down the information to be provided into smaller chunks
- Pause to check for understanding after delivering a chunk of information.

Teach back:

- The onus for the paediatric patient's and caregiver's understanding is on the nurse
- Explain clearly and check understanding by asking the paediatric patient and their caregiver to teach back to you what they have learned
- Do not ask 'Do you understand?'
- Ask something similar to 'I'd like to check I've explained things clearly. Can you please explain back to me what this medication is for?'
- Use open-ended, non-shaming questions
- Allow the paediatric patient and their caregiver to explain in their own words
- If necessary, 're-teach', that is explain again in a different way and re-check understanding
- A different learning modality or more time may be needed for the 're-teach'.

This online learning module (http://teachback.org/) has been developed to support health professionals in Australia to use teach-back in their practice.

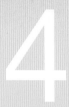

CHAPTER 4

Administration considerations for the paediatric patient

Rinnah Peacock, Kerry Reid-Searl, Pauline Davies

Cognitive considerations

Assessing the developmental level of the paediatric patient is important to establish their level of understanding and cooperation as discussed in Chapter 3. Once medications are ready for administering, the nurse can then implement age-appropriate strategies (Table 4.1).

Administering medication to a paediatric patient requires effective communication. Age-appropriate language should be employed.

Respectful, clear and professional communication is also paramount in establishing a positive relationship with the caregiver.

Box 4.1 highlights some tips for gaining cooperation with the paediatric patient with a focus on communication.

TABLE 4.1 Age-appropriate strategies to promote medication administration

AGE	STRATEGY
Infant	Assistance with significant other and appropriate holding

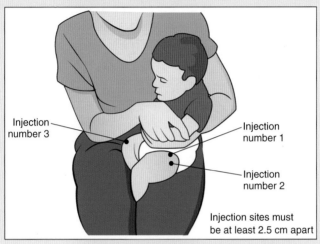

Injection number 3

Injection number 1

Injection number 2

Injection sites must be at least 2.5 cm apart

Parent cuddling the patient, while administering IM injection in the leg (Source: Australian Technical Advisory Group on Immunisation [ATAGI]. Australian Immunisation Handbook, Australian Government Department of Health and Aged Care, Canberra, 2024. https://immunisationhandbook.health.gov.au/ resources/figures/figure-recommended-technique-for-giving-multiple-vaccine-injections-into-the-antero-lateral-thigh-in-an-infant. Date accessed: 12 January 2024. © 2024 Commonwealth of Australia as represented by the Department of Health and Aged Care.)

Toddler	Negotiation with distraction, games and reward For example, get down close to the child's face and energetically sing a song – while another nurse performs the procedure

Continued

TABLE 4.1   Age-appropriate strategies to promote
medication administration   *continued*

Preschool	Negotiation with distraction, games and reward Use distraction toys – toys that require the child's participation (e.g., blow toys or bubbles) often work best for this age group

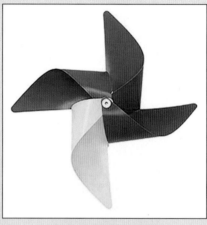

School age	Promote independence, clear instruction, games and reward A reward example would be when a child can select a gift of their choosing from the 'reward box' on the successful completion of the task
Adolescent	Promote independence, clear instruction The patient may be able to complete the procedure on a mannequin first or may be able to independently complete aspects of the procedure (e.g., remove the numbing cream from site, prior to injection)

Involving caregivers at the point of administration

Involving the caregiver can provide comfort for the paediatric patient. Questions to consider with caregiver involvement include:

- Do they have the capacity to assist effectively in the administration?
  - If not consider supportive strategies.

Box 4.1 **Tips for gaining rapport and cooperation with the paediatric patient**	
R	**R**espectful, warm and open greeting to the child and the parent/caregiver
A	**A**dvise the child and the parent/caregiver about the procedure ensuring you take time to determine what their understanding is of the medication. This includes the reasons for taking the medication, the actions, side effects and how to take it
P	**P**repare to negotiate in gaining cooperation for administration, e.g., if the child wants to self-administer and/or the parent/caregiver wants to assist. Show the parent/caregiver how they can assist, e.g., holding the child, where to stand in line with the child's vision, or using a distraction toy, etc.
P	**P**lan for distraction techniques if necessary, i.e., a book, computer game, toy, puppet etc. Let the child know what they can do during the administration; e.g., if an IMI they could count out loud, squeeze a doll/ teddy, squeeze a hand, etc.
O	**O**pen communication using concrete terms and age-appropriate words that the child and parent/caregiver can understand. In the communication, be honest with the child. For example, tell the child what the medication may taste like or if the injection will sting, what the IV injection may feel like and how long it will take to deliver
R	**R**eward. Consider what the outcome might be for the child in negotiation with the parent/caregiver if they are cooperative in taking the medication. For example, game time, a sticker, etc.
T	**T**ell the child and parent/caregiver what they will feel like after taking the medication, e.g., if it will relieve pain or stop nausea

- Do they understand why the paediatric patient requires the medication and via what route?
  - If not, provide clear explanation prior to the procedure.
- Do they want to be present?
  - If so, give clear instruction of how they can help support the paediatric patient. If they do not want to be present, provide instruction on where they can wait.

- Are they willing to hold the paediatric patient in a way that assists the nurse to administer medication safely?
    - If so, provide a demonstration and clear instructions. If not, explain what will occur and where they can be best positioned during the procedure.

When administering medication, consider age-appropriate distraction strategies (Box 4.2 and Fig. 4.1).

Environment

The environment must be appropriate for the paediatric patient, caregiver and nurse when administering medications to the paediatric patient. Considerations include:

- Is the area a safe space?
    - Some medications can be given at the bedside, for example, oral or intravenous (IV); however, others, such as intramuscular injection (IMI) or rectal, may be traumatic for the paediatric patient and a safe space needs to be created away from the bedside.

Box 4.2 **Examples of strategies for distraction**	
All ages (make sure there are a variety of resources so age-appropriate selection can occur)	Toys, books, sensory and tactile toys
School-age children	Computer or iPhone resources (some caregivers may not allow children to use phones: ask for consent from caregivers prior to suggesting)
School-age children (works best with children that play computer games and are used to this technology)	Virtual reality
All children (be aware that some children may have a fear associated with puppets)	Puppets/role play
All ages (do not assume that older children do not want to hold their parent's hand)	Other person to play, hold or listen to during the administration

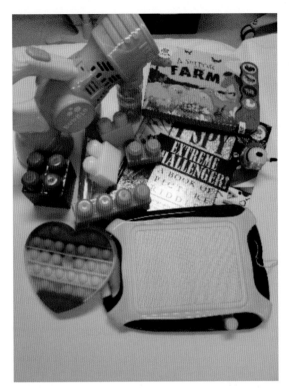

Figure 4.1 Examples of resources used for distraction.

- Is there a safe working area?
  - Consider bed height, area being free from clutter, limited guests/visitors, sufficient lighting.
- Are there other people around?
  - Siblings (or other patients) can become upset if witness to procedure.
- Does your hospital have access to a Play Therapist?
  - Provide an experienced person to assist with distraction techniques.
- Are there distraction resources available?
  - Setting these up and getting patient used to distraction tools prior can be beneficial.

The paediatric patient who refuses medication

It is acceptable for the paediatric patient or their caregiver to refuse medications. Sometimes the refusal is due to lack of knowledge or education in relation to the need or requirement of specific medication. Sometimes caregivers do not want to go through the perceived or real trauma of administering the medication. Good education and preparation of the paediatric patient and caregiver is essential.

In some circumstances, the paediatric patient may still refuse but the need for taking the medication is in the best interest of the paediatric patient. For these circumstances some strategies to assist may include:

- The patient may need to be held (see use of restraint below). If so, encourage the caregiver to do the holding. The paediatric patient should be advised that holding is not about punishment but rather the need for them to have the medication and again explain importance.
- If holding, this should be in a position of comfort in a semi-reclined position.
- To hold the paediatric patient the caregiver or nurse can position them on their lap with the paediatric patient's right arm behind them. The left hand of the paediatric patient can then be held and their head can be securely positioned between the holder's arm and body (as seen in Fig. 4.2).

When administering oral medication, it is important NOT to deliver medication to the paediatric patient who is lying flat and screaming as this increases the chance of aspiration (adapted from Anderson & Herring 2019).

Use of holding and restraint

Ideally medication is administered to the paediatric patient without the need to hold them. However, infants and young children may differ. If holding is required, this must be discussed with caregivers and consent obtained. For organisations that use seclusion/restraint (outside of physical holding) for children and youth, the seclusion/restraint standards apply. Nurses should always adhere to organisational policy. This is often used only if

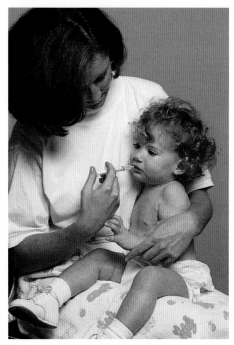

Figure 4.2 A nurse partially restrains a child for easy and comfortable administration of oral medication. (Hockenberry et al 2019.)

all other methods have been exhausted as this can result in the child becoming quite distressed. Sometimes it is the only way that essential medication can be administered to paediatric patients. Debrief with the child, their parents and staff involved afterwards as seeing this could be traumatic for all involved.

5

Practising safely

Kerry Reid-Searl, Pauline Davies, Rinnah Peacock

The role of the nurse in preparing and administering medications

When administering medications to the paediatric patient, safety is a priority. The nurse requires:

- Knowledge of the physiological differences among children compared with adults in relation to medications in total (e.g., dosage, effect, absorption, administration)
- Knowledge about medications and how to access information
- Knowledge of different drug types and actions
- An understanding of medication charts and the medication order
- Knowledge of routes for administration
- An ability to practise safe administration principles.

Getting started

Before the nurse undertakes preparation of medications, they need to undertake a self-assessment and ask:

- Am I tired, hungry, late, free of distraction?
    - If yes address these prior to preparing the medication.
- Is there the correct number of appropriately qualified nurses present to check and prepare the medication?
    - When administering medications to a paediatric patient, double-checking must occur and should be an independent cognitive task, meaning the nurse independently calculates the amount required rather than checking or glancing at someone else's calculations. The double-checking should commence from the point of preparing the drug and should continue to the point of administration. Double-checking is central to patient safety and reducing drug errors (Ramasamy et al 2013).
- Is the environment free of distractions?
    - When preparing medications avoid conversations with others unless specific to the preparation process. Try to be in a quiet non-interrupted space and advise peers that you are preparing medications and do not want interruptions.
- Is the area clean?
    - See Figure 5.1 for an example of a clean working area.

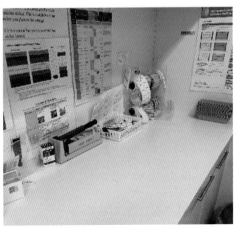

Figure 5.1 A clean working area.

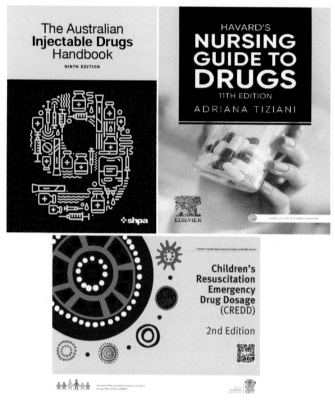

Figure 5.2 Resources for checking medication.

- Are there appropriate resources and equipment accessible?
  - For example, Medication Information Resources, either hard copy or online (Fig. 5.2), and appropriate administration equipment, e.g., oral syringes (see Fig. 5.10).

Before getting started the nurse should be cognisant of the safety checks that will be required in preparation and delivery.

The next part of this guide introduces the safety checks.

A reminder of safety checks

The safety checks encompass the six rights of medication (Fig. 5.3). The checks more broadly include:

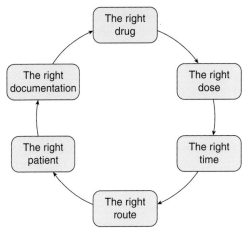

Figure 5.3 The six rights of medication administration.

CHECK THE ORDER: DRUG NAME, DOSE, TIME, ROUTE, FREQUENCY

Check that the information, drug name (preferably generic rather than trade name), dose utilising the appropriate resources, route, frequency, time due and when the drug was last given are all legible and that the order is signed by the medical officer. If any doubt exists, withhold the drug and check with the medical officer.

CHECK THE MEDICATION

- Check that a second appropriately qualified nurse is present.
- Check the container label against the medication order when selecting the preparation, before measuring out and when replacing the preparation.
- Check the expiry date of the drug.
- Complete the drug calculation and then check the answer with another appropriately qualified nurse, a pharmacist or medical officer (ask the second person to do the calculation independently, then compare answers). Remember that when administering medications in the paediatric population the amount of drug will differ to adults and to check drug preparations (e.g. do not quarter a 200 mg tablet if 50 mg tablet is available) half a tablet or more than two tablets or one ampoule at a time.

- Mix liquid contents thoroughly but rotate or swirl protein preparations gently to prevent denaturation and frothing. If the reconstituted solution containing protein is further diluted, it should be gently inverted (not shaken) to ensure even mixing.
- Do not over-handle tablets.
- Note any discolouration, precipitate or foreign bodies (do not administer if they are present).
- Once the medication is prepared, the appropriately qualified nurse must complete the appropriate labelling as required within the organisation. Example of labelling is included in the below section on intravenous (IV) medications.

CHECK THE PATIENT

- Check that the paediatric patient details are correct, including any known allergies. It is important to discuss any allergy/sensitivity history with the paediatric patient and/or caregiver as cross-sensitivity between products does occur.
- Check the paediatric patient identity carefully (check wrist identity band or verbally), taking extra care if there are children with the same or similar names, or if the paediatric patient is unknown to the nurse.
- Check that the paediatric patient and caregiver know the reason for the medication and discuss any query with the medical officer before giving the medication.

DOCUMENTATION

- Ensure that the drug administration chart is signed after administration.
- Document any discrepancies (e.g., patient unable or refuses to take medication, patient absent, medication not available).
- If Schedule 8 medications are involved, ensure that the drug register is correctly filled in (date, time, patient, drug [form, strength, amount to be administered], persons administering drug, balance of drug remaining, any drug discarded).
- Observe the paediatric patient and document in the patient's history and note beneficial effects and/or report and chart any adverse effects (see Box 5.1).

> **Box 5.1**
> **Effects of medications: general tips**
>
> A medication may produce more than one effect, which may be beneficial or not
> - The *desired action* is the physiological response the medication is expected to cause (e.g., pain relief medications are expected to reduce pain)
> - An *adverse effect* refers to an unwanted effect, which may or may not be dose related and is usually via a different mechanism to its pharmacological action
> - *Toxic effects* develop after prolonged administration of high doses of medication, or when a medication accumulates in the blood because of impaired metabolism or excretion
> - *Allergic reactions* are unpredictable responses to a medication that acts as an antigen, triggering the release of antibodies. Allergic reactions may be mild (such as urticaria [hives] and pruritus [itching]), or they may be severe (e.g., severe wheezing and respiratory distress), or life threatening (e.g., anaphylactic reaction). Some reactions occur within minutes of the drug being given (e.g., penicillin, streptomycin, radiological contrast media), while other allergic reactions may be delayed for hours or days (e.g., contact sensitivity to local anaesthetic cream)
> - *Idiosyncratic reactions* are those where the paediatric patient's body either overreacts or underreacts to a medication, or when the reaction is unusual and there is no known cause (e.g., the antihistamine promethazine [Phenergan] is sometimes used for sedation; however, in some people [especially children] it can cause insomnia and agitation)
> - *Pharmacogenetic reactions* occur because a paediatric patient may have a genetic trait that leads to abnormal reactions to medications
> - *Drug tolerance* may also occur where a paediatric patient has a decreased response to a drug over time, necessitating an increase in dosage to achieve the required response (Bryant et al 2019)
> - *Drug interactions* occur when one drug modifies the action of another drug (e.g., a drug may either increase or decrease the action of other medications). A drug interaction may be synergistic (enhances the effects of another drug), antagonistic (opposes the effects of another drug) or additive (where the two drug actions are added together)

DRUG EFFECTS

Check the effect of the medication on the paediatric patient (Box 5.1).

General tips

- Never administer a medication if the order is unclear or incomplete
- Always work out the expected drug dosage per weight of the paediatric patient and double-check with an appropriately qualified nurse
- Always question drug dosages if they do not fall in the recommended dosage for weight
- Do not rely on caregiver estimates of weight, instead weigh the paediatric patient on suitable scales
- Always check allergies prior to administration
- Only give medications that you, the appropriately qualified nurse, have prepared
- Never leave medications on bedside tables, lockers or dinner trays
- Wait until oral medications are swallowed
- If you are a student, always seek direct supervision from the point of preparation to administration

While the safety checks have been introduced, the next part of this guide elaborates on some sections of the checking.

DISPOSAL

Correctly and safely dispose of equipment at point of use; return whole unused medications to pharmacy (e.g., do not recap syringes, dispose of them safely in a sharps container; return unused medications to pharmacy).

Knowledge about medications and accessing information

It is a legal responsibility that nurses have knowledge about the medications they are administering. This includes drug class, purpose, action, recommended and usual dose range, how it is administered, contraindications, side effects, allergic reactions (including food and other medication incompatibility).

Nurses are not expected to memorise all this information, but they do need to know where to access the appropriate information prior to administration. Once a nurse has knowledge then they must question and act upon any unclear order, assess what skills are required to carry out the order and understand what to observe for in terms of beneficial and adverse effects (Harvard xvii Tiziani 2021).

Examples of resources include (see Fig. 5.2):

- The *AMH Children's Dosing Companion* and the *Australian Injectable Drugs Handbook*
- The *PIG Drug Guidelines* (Lilley et al 2019)
- MIMS Online
- *Children's Resuscitation Emergency Drug Dosage* (CREDD).

MEDICATION TYPES AND ACTIONS

There are many different types of medications with varying actions. The nurse should always refer to medication resources to determine the action of any drug before administering.

Table 5.1 includes common types of medications and their actions.

High-risk medications

Some medications require high levels of caution with administration. APINCHS medications (Table 5.2) are those that are known to have a high risk of medication-related harm. Any medications within these categories must be double-checked with two qualified persons in preparation and administration. These are medications that nurses must be especially vigilant about as the consequence of errors can cause significant harm to the patient.

Understanding charts and the medication order

In preparing to administer medication, the nurse should understand the paediatric medication order and what constitutes an order. To appreciate what is included in an order, it is necessary to first consider the paediatric-specific medication chart.

MEDICATION CHARTS

In Australia there is the Paediatric National Inpatient Medication Chart (NIMC). This chart is used when caring for children who are inpatients in a healthcare facility (Fig. 5.4).

TABLE 5.1 Different medication types and general action

COMMON TYPES OF MEDICATION	ACTION
Antibiotic	Disrupts essential processes or structures in the bacterial cell either killing or slowing down bacterial growth
Analgesic	Relieves pain
Aperient	Any oral agent that promotes the expulsion of faeces, including harsh stimulant laxatives, saline laxatives, stool softeners, bulking laxatives and lubricants
Anti-emetic	Medication used to treat nausea and vomiting
Anti-convulsant/ Anti-epileptic	Helps normalise the way nerve impulses travel along the nerve cells, which helps prevent or treat seizures
Bronchodilator	Makes breathing easier by relaxing the muscles in the lungs and widening the airway
Chemotherapy	Damages the gene inside the nucleus of the cell. The medication targets cells at different stages of the cell cycle
Insulin	Pharmaceutical preparation of the protein hormone insulin that is used to treat high blood glucose
Non-steroidal anti-inflammatory (NSAID)	Reduces inflammation (redness, swelling and pain)
Opioid	A broad group of pain-relieving medication that works by interacting with opioid receptors in body cells to muffle the perception of pain and boost feelings of pleasure

Source: Tiziani (2020) Havard's Nursing Guide to Drugs.

All medication charts must include:
- The patient details with a current patient identification label or at a minimum:
  - patient name, UR number, date of birth and gender written in legible print
  - weight and height (Fig. 5.5)
  - allergies and adverse reactions (ADR).

TABLE 5.2 APINCHS medication

A	Antimicrobials	Aminoglycosides: gentamicin, tobramycin and amikacin vancomycin amphotericin – liposomal formulation
P	Potassium and other electrolytes	Injections of concentrated electrolytes: potassium magnesium calcium hypertonic sodium chloride
I	Insulin	All insulins
N	Narcotics (opioids) and other sedatives	Hydromorphone oxycodone Morphine Fentanyl Alfentanil Remifentanil Analgesic patches Diazepam Midazolam Thiopentone Propofol Other short-term anaesthetics
C	Chemotherapeutic Agents	Vincristine Methotrexate Etoposide Azathioprine Oral chemotherapy
H	Heparin and other anticoagulants	Heparin and low molecular weight heparins (LMWH): dalteparin enoxaparin Warfarin Direct oral anticoagulants (DOACs): dabigatran rivaroxaban apixaban
S	Systems	Medication safety systems such as: independent double-checks safe administration of liquid medications standardised order sets medication charts

Australian Commission on Safety and Quality in Health Care (2022) APINCHS classification of high risk medicines. Accessed 14 March 2024.

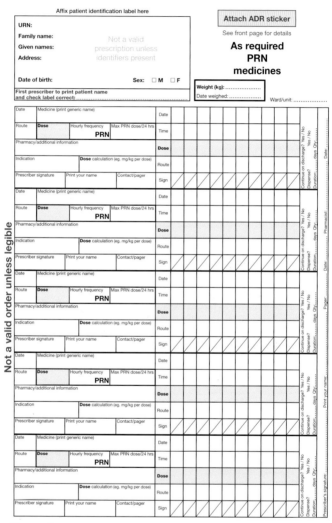

Figure 5.4 National Inpatient Medication Chart (NIMC) – Paediatric.
Reproduced with permission from National Inpatient Medication Chart
(NIMC) - Paediatric, developed by the Australian Commission on Safety
and Quality in Health Care (ACSQHC). ACSQHC: Sydney 2012.

Cut off section

⚕ Paediatric Medication chart number .... of ....

Facility/service:..

Ward/unit:..

Additional charts
☐ IV fluid   ☐ BGL/insulin   ☐ Acute pain   ☐ IV heparin
☐ Inhalation   ☐ Palliative care   ☐ Chemotherapy   ☐ Other

Once only medicines

Date prescribed	Medicine (print generic name)	Route	Dose	Dose calc eg. mg/kg per dose	Date/time to be given	Prescriber Signature	Print your name	Given by	Date/time given	Pharm

Telephone orders (to be signed within 24 hours of order)

Date time	Medicine (print generic name)	Route	Dose	Dose calc eg. mg/kg per Dose	Frequency	Check initials N1	N2	Prescriber name	Pres. sign	Date	Record of administration Time / given by	Time / given by	Time / given by

Medicines taken prior to presentation to hospital
(prescribed, over the counter, complementary)   Own medicines brought in? ☐ Y ☐ N

Medicine and formulation	Dose and frequency	Duration	Medicine and formulation	Dose and frequency	Duration

Not for administration

GP:	Community pharmacy:
Sign: Print: Date:	Medicines usually administered by:

DO NOT WRITE IN THIS BINDING MARGIN

⚕ Paediatric

NIMC (paediatric)

⚕ Paediatric

© Commonwealth of Australia 2005 – As amended 2019

Continued

Cut off section

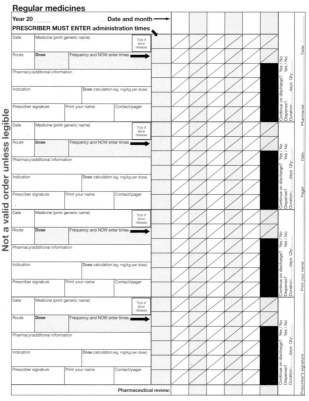

Figure 5.4, *continued*

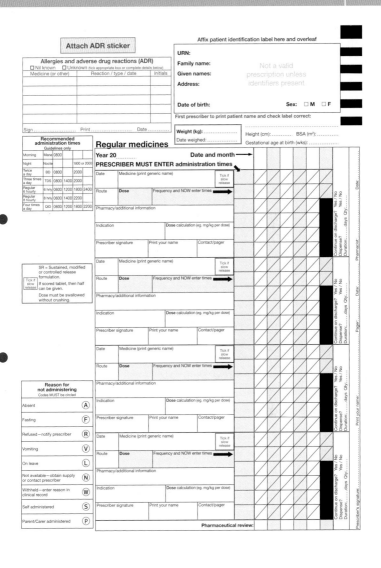

Attach ADR sticker

Allergies and adverse drug reactions (ADR)
☐ Nil known ☐ Unknown (tick appropriate box or complete details below)

Medicine (or other)	Reaction / type / date	Initials

Sign .... Print .... Date ....

Affix patient identification label here and overleaf

URN:

Family name:

Given names:

Address:

Not a valid prescription unless identifiers present

Date of birth: Sex: ☐ M ☐ F

First prescriber to print patient name and check label correct:

Weight (kg): ....
Date weighed: ....

Height (cm): .... BSA (m²): ....
Gestational age at birth (wks): ....

Recommended administration times
Guidelines only

Morning	Mane	0800		
Night	Nocte		1800 or 2000	
Twice a day	BD	0800	2000	
Three times a day	TDS	0800	1400	2000
Regular 6 hourly	6 hrly	0600	1200	1800	2400
Regular 8 hourly	8 hrly	0600	1400	2200	
Four times a day	QID	0600	1200	1800	2200

Regular medicines

Year 20 ____
PRESCRIBER MUST ENTER administration times
Date and month ➡

SR = Sustained, modified or controlled release formulation.

Tick if slow release If scored tablet, then half can be given.

Dose must be swallowed without crushing.

Reason for not administering
Codes MUST be circled

Absent	Ⓐ
Fasting	Ⓕ
Refused—notify prescriber	Ⓡ
Vomiting	Ⓥ
On leave	Ⓛ
Not available—obtain supply or contact prescriber	Ⓝ
Withheld—enter reason in clinical record	Ⓦ
Self administered	Ⓢ
Parent/Carer administered	Ⓟ

Date | Medicine (print generic name) | Tick if slow release
Route | **Dose** | Frequency and NOW enter times ➡
Pharmacy/additional information
Indication | Dose calculation (eg. mg/kg per dose)
Prescriber signature | Print your name | Contact/pager

Pharmaceutical review:

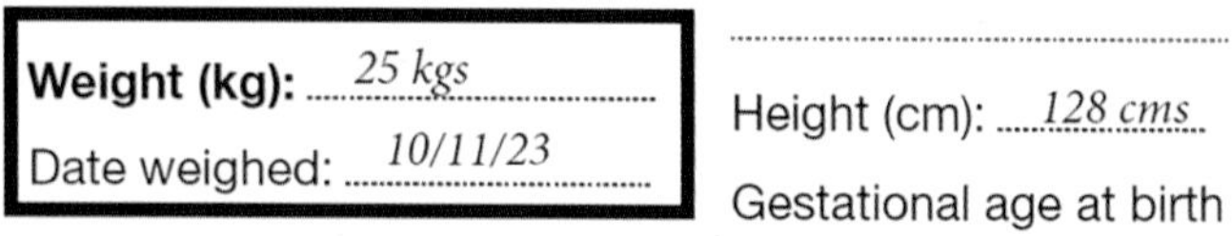

Weight (kg):	_25 kgs_
Date weighed:	_10/11/23_

Height (cm): _128 cms_

Gestational age at birth

Figure 5.5 Weight and height.

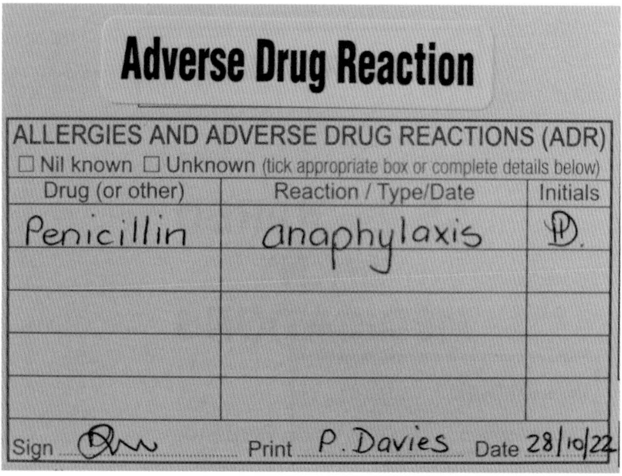

Adverse Drug Reaction

ALLERGIES AND ADVERSE DRUG REACTIONS (ADR)		
☐ Nil known ☐ Unknown (tick appropriate box or complete details below)		
Drug (or other)	Reaction / Type/Date	Initials
Penicillin	anaphylaxis	P.
Sign ___	Print P. Davies	Date 28/10/22

Figure 5.6 Allergy documented and alert sticker in place.

If the patient has an allergy, the following must be completed in the appropriate section:

- Name of drug/substance documented
- Reaction details documented
- Date that the reaction occurred documented
- Alert and ADR stickers affixed to the front and back of the paediatric NIMC (Fig. 5.6)
- Drug allergy alert ID band attached to the patient.

THE MEDICATION ORDER

The order is valid only if the prescribing medical officer enters all the listed items as follow (Fig. 5.7):

- Patient details
- Allergy
- Date

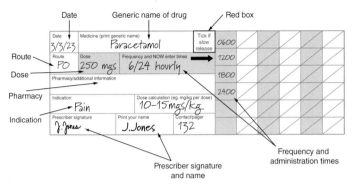

Figure 5.7 Elements of valid order.

- Generic drug name
- The red tick if slow-release box
- Route
- Dose
- Frequency and administration times
- Pharmacy
- Indication
- Doctor's signature and printed name.

Also check when the medication was last given. If any doubt withhold administration and check with the medical officer. When checking a valid order, it is vital that the nurse has knowledge of the different forms of medications and understands the meanings of abbreviations for routes and times. Table 5.3 highlights commonly used forms of medication.

There are commonly used and understood abbreviations for routes and dose (Table 5.4 & see Table 1.3), and there are commonly used and understood abbreviations for times (Table 5.5). There are recommended administration times as a guideline only (Table 5.6).

The medication label

The medication label (Fig. 5.8) should contain:
- The generic and trade name of the medication
- The active ingredients in the medication
- The form of the medication
- The approved route for administration

TABLE 5.3   Forms of medication and description

FORM	MEANING
Tablet	Tablet for oral administration
Capsule	Gelatine cover, either hard or soft, encapsulating the medication for oral administration
Sprinkles	Medications containing pellets or granules that can be mixed with food for oral administration
Elixir	Liquid form of medication for oral administration
Ung/topical	Ointment for skin surface
Suppository	A solid medical preparation either conical or cylindrical designed for vaginal or rectal insertion
Injection	A liquid medication designed for intramuscular, subcutaneous, IV administration
Inhalation	A medication prepared to be delivered in the form of vapour or spray
Eye drop	Liquid medication administered onto the surface of the eye

TABLE 5.4   Abbreviations for routes for medication administration

ROUTE ABBREVIATION	MEANING
CVC	Central venous catheter
PO	Per oral: via the mouth
IV	Intravenous: into the vein via an IV cannula
IM	Intramuscular: into the muscle via injection
Intranasal	Via the nose
MA	Metered aerosol
Neb	Nebulised/nebuliser
SC	Subcutaneous: under the skin and into SC tissue via injection
SL	Sublingual: under the tongue
TOPICAL	Topical: on the skin
PR	Per rectal: via the anus

TABLE 5.4 Abbreviations for routes for medication administration   *continued*

ROUTE ABBREVIATION	MEANING
PEG	Percutaneous endoscopic gastrostomy
PICC	Peripheral inserted central catheter
NGT	Nasogastric: via the nose into the stomach
IO	Intraosseous: into the bone via a cannula
PV	Per vagina

TABLE 5.5 Abbreviations for times and meaning

ABBREVIATION	MEANING
mane	Morning
nocte	Night
bd	Twice daily
tds	Three times a day
qid	Four times a day
unit(s)	International Unit(s)

Reproduced with permission from Recommendations for terminology, abbreviations and symbols used in medicines documentation - Summary sheet, developed by the Australian Commission on Safety and Quality in Health Care (ACSQHC). ACSQHC: Sydney 2016.

- The manufacturer of the drug
- The strength in stock
- The quantity in stock
- The poisons schedule
- The batch number
- The expiry date.

Nursing alert

A nurse should not proceed to administer medication if the medication order is not complete, if the handwriting is illegible, if it is not printed, if part of the order has been erased or whiteout has been used. If apparent, the order should be rewritten.

TABLE 5.6	Recommended administration times				
MEANING	ABBREVIATION	TIME			
Night	nocte			1800 or 2000	
Twice a day	bd	0800		2000	
Three times a day	tds	0800	1400	2000	
Antibiotic	6-hourly	0600	1200	1800	2400
Antibiotic	8-hourly	0600	1400	2200	
Four times per day	qid	0600	1200	1800	2200

Reproduced with permission from National Inpatient Medication Chart (NIMC) - Paediatric, developed by the Australian Commission on Safety and Quality in Health Care (ACSQHC). ACSQHC: Sydney 2012.

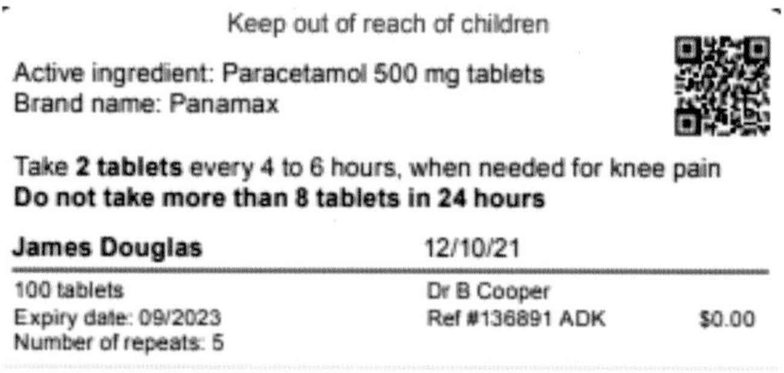

Keep out of reach of children

Active ingredient: Paracetamol 500 mg tablets
Brand name: Panamax

Take **2 tablets** every 4 to 6 hours, when needed for knee pain
Do not take more than 8 tablets in 24 hours

James Douglas	12/10/21	
100 tablets	Dr B Cooper	
Expiry date: 09/2023	Ref #136891 ADK	$0.00
Number of repeats: 5		

Figure 5.8 Medication label.

Telephone orders

If the nurse caring for the paediatric patient receives a telephone order (Fig. 5.9) for the medication, the following must be documented in the appropriate section of the chart:

- Date prescribed
- Generic name of medicine
- Route of administration
- Dose to be administered
- Frequency medicine is to be administered

Date prescribed

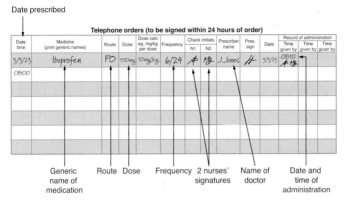

Figure 5.9 Telephone order.

- Initials of two appropriately qualified nurses to confirm the verbal order heard and double-checked
- Name of doctor giving verbal order
- Time of administration
- Initials of person who administers the medicine
- Prescription explanation (abbreviations, terminology, times, legal requirements, allergies, electronic prescribing, standing orders).

Routes for medication administration

In preparing medications the nurse must know the required route. Table 5.4 provides an abbreviation and the meaning for each route. The next section explores the most common routes for the paediatric patient.

ORAL MEDICATIONS

Oral medications are the most common form of medication administration for paediatric patients. This can be in the form of a tablet, an elixir, a capsule or sprinkles.

The nurse needs to understand the specific requirements of the oral medication. For example:

- Can it be given with food?
- Is there a timeframe in which it needs to be given prior to or after food?

- Can it be crushed?
- Must it be swallowed whole and not chewed?
- Can it be given with yoghurt or apple juice?
- Can it be given with other medications?

> **Nursing alert**
>
> A great resource to check if medications can or cannot be crushed is *Don't Rush to Crush* (https://www.mims.com.au/newsletter/201304/Crush.pdf).

The nurse needs to know and adhere to the manufacturer's recommendations to avoid the following:
- Altered absorption
- Instability of the medication
- Local irritation
- Medication not reaching the intended site
- Unfavourable tastes
- Hazardous effects.

It is important to consider age variations in oral administration. Perhaps the most challenging is the infant and younger paediatric patient. Consider the following when administering oral medications to this cohort.

The infant
- Caution must be given in the way the infant is positioned to prevent aspiration.
- The infant should be held in a semi-reclined position.
- A caregiver can be of assistance in holding the infant – see Use of holding and restraint in Chapter 4.
- A disposable oral calibrated syringe should be used for liquids and the medication can be delivered along the side of the infant's tongue. The medication should be administered slowly and in small amounts. The nurse should wait until the infant swallows before administering any further volume.
- Medication may need to be retrieved from the lips or chin and re-fed to the infant.
- If the infant is breastfeeding, the syringe can be placed into the side of the mouth, parallel to the nipple. The medication can be delivered while the infant breastfeeds.

- Medication should not be added to the infant's formula because the infant may not take all the formula. (Adapted from Anderson & Herring 2019.)

The toddler/child

- Oral medications are available in a variety of forms, including tablets (solid, chewable or dissolving), capsules, sprinkles and oral mixtures.
- The nurse needs to determine the paediatric patient's ability to swallow oral medications. This will be influenced by developmental age, size of the paediatric patient and the paediatric patient's past experiences.
- Oral mixtures can be unpleasant to taste and may need to be camouflaged with an appropriate solution, for example, syrup, honey.
- Disposable oral calibrated syringes are the preferred device for dosing accuracy in oral mixtures. It is important for safety reasons to use specifically designed oral syringes. These should not be compatible with needles or IV access. These are orange in colour (Fig. 5.10).
- Paper cups are not suitable for oral mixtures, instead use a plastic cup with clearly defined markers (Fig. 5.11)
  - teaspoons are not an accurate measuring device and are subject to error.

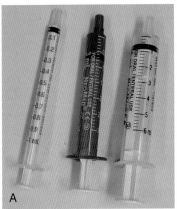
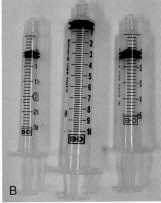

Figure 5.10 Oral syringes (a) and IV syringes (b).

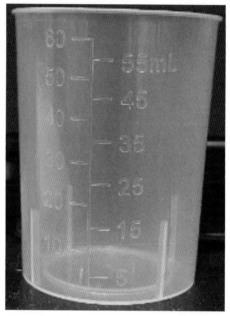

Figure 5.11 An appropriate plastic cup for oral administration of medication.

- The dropper is also an unreliable device for measuring oral mixtures. Viscous liquids produce larger drops than thin liquids. In general, a dropper is not used as a device for measuring medication unless the device is specific and comes with the medication.
- Some children have trouble swallowing oral tablets. If the medication is not available in mixture/liquid form, then the medication may need to be crushed. However, confirmation must be made to see if it can be crushed. (Check resource: *Don't Rush to Crush* [https://www.mims.com.au/newsletter/201304/Crush.pdf]).
- If able to crush the medication, a crushing device should be used.
- Some crushed medications can be mixed with an appropriate solution, for example, syrup, honey.
  (Adapted from Anderson & Herring 2019.)
  Also see Box 5.2.

Box 5.2
General tips in administering oral medication

- Try to obtain the paediatric patient's cooperation
- Give choices to the paediatric patient – they may want to push the oral syringe plunger
- Give the paediatric patient some options in negotiation – they may want to take it at the completion of an activity, negotiate a game, such as giving a doll or teddy and the medication at the same time, or they may be rewarded with a game after taking the medication
- Establish some strategies that work for the paediatric patient to take the medication, i.e., pinching their nose, etc.
- Where able, camouflage the medication with an appropriate amount of sweet-tasting substance
- When delivering the medication, do so in small amounts/increments and allow the paediatric patient to swallow between squirts
- Place the syringe in the corner pocket of the paediatric patient's mouth between the lower teeth and cheek
- Do not aim for the back of the throat or administer while the paediatric patient is lying down – this increases the risk of aspiration
- Be prepared with a drink following the medication – note that dairy products may impact on absorption of the medication

Nursing alert

If a paediatric patient vomits or spits medication out, do not readminister – instead contact the medical officer and seek advice. There are many considerations including how much the paediatric patient vomited or spat out and the timing of it from the point of administration.
   *When the nurse administers oral medication to a paediatric patient where there is risk that they could vomit or spit, the nurse should don personal protective equipment (PPE) and, specifically, mask and eye protection.
   To gain further understanding of oral administration of medication, refer to Paediatric skill 7.3 in Chapter 7.

INTRAMUSCULAR MEDICATIONS

The volume of medication ordered for an intramuscular (IM) injection for the paediatric patient requires the selection of a syringe that enables accurate measurement of small amounts of solution. For volumes less than 1 mL, syringes calibrated in

0.01-mL increments are appropriate whereas for volumes less than 0.5 mL, a 0.5-mL syringe is ideal. These low-dose syringes with the appropriate needles minimise the chance of administering incorrect amounts because of dead space. Dead space allows fluid to remain in the syringe after the plunger is pushed completely to the end of the syringe. A minimum of 0.2 mL can remain in the syringe with dead space in a standard needle hub (Anderson & Herring 2019).

See Figure 5.12 for an image of different sizes of syringes. Figure 5.13 illustrates the various parts of a syringe.

When choosing a needle for an IM injection, it must be long enough to penetrate through the subcutaneous tissue and deposit the medication into muscle. The needles causing least discomfort are 25–30 gauge; however, if the solution is viscous, a larger gauge may be needed (also see Fig. 5.14).

The two main muscles used for IM injections are:

- The lateral aspect of the thigh (middle third when the thigh is divided into three; Fig. 5.15)
- The deltoid (Fig. 5.16).

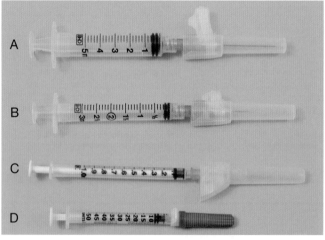

Figure 5.12 Types of syringes. (a) 5-mL syringe (Luer lock). (b) 3-mL syringe (Luer lock). (c) Tuberculin syringe marked in 0.01-mm (hundredths) increments for doses < 1 mL. (d) Insulin syringe marked in units (50). (Crisp et al 2013.)

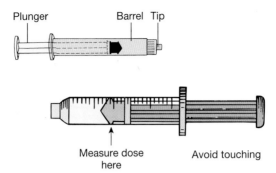

Figure 5.13 Parts of a syringe. (Crisp et al 2013.)

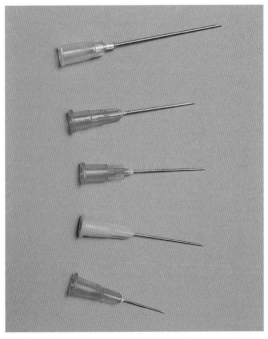

Figure 5.14 Syringe needles. Top to bottom: 19 gauge, 38-mm length; 20 gauge, 25-mm length; 21 gauge, 25-mm length; 23 gauge, 25-mm length; and 25 gauge, 16-mm length. (Crisp et al 2013.)

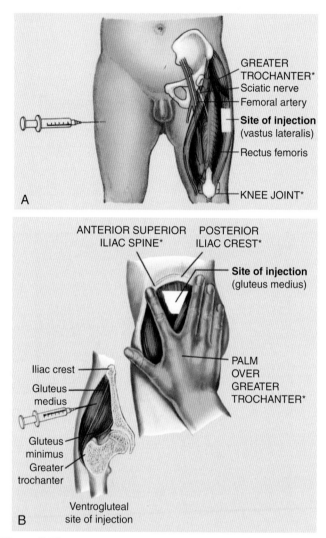

Figure 5.15 Injection sites in children. **(a)** Vastus lateralis.
(b) Ventrogluteal. (Hockenberry et al 2019.)

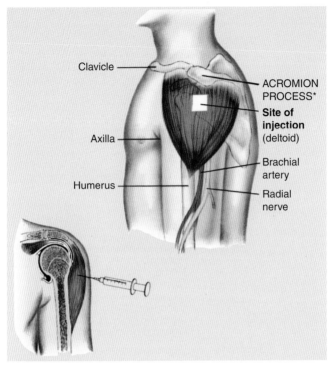

Figure 5.16 Injection site in children (deltoid). (Hockenberry et al 2019.)

No more than 5 mL should be administered by IM injection, and less into the deltoid muscle. If a volume greater than 5 mL is required, the dose should be divided and given into different sites.

For more details see Table 5.7. This includes location, needle insertion and size, advantages and disadvantages.

Determining the site for an IM injection

There are several factors to consider when deciding the best site for an IM injection in the paediatric patient. These include:

- The amount of medication to be given (usually 1 mL is the maximum volume that should be administered into a single muscle site in a small paediatric patient or infant). It should be noted that the muscle mass of small infants may not tolerate more than 0.5 mL of volume.

TABLE 5.7   Intramuscular injection sites in children

	VASTUS LATERALIS (see Fig. 5.16a)	VENTROGLUTEAL (see Fig. 5.16b)	DELTOID (see Fig. 5.17)
Location*	Palpate to find greater trochanter and knee joints; divide vertical distance between these two landmarks into thirds; inject into middle third	Palpate to locate greater trochanter, anterior superior iliac tubercle (found by flexing thigh at hip and measuring up to 1–2 cm [0.4–0.8 inch] above crease formed in groin), and posterior iliac crest; place palm of hand over greater trochanter, index finger over anterior superior iliac tubercle, and middle finger along crest of ileum posteriorly as far as possible; inject into centre of V formed by fingers	Locate acromion process; inject only into upper third of muscle that begins about two finger-widths below acromion
Needle insertion and size	Insert needle perpendicular to knee in infants and young children, or perpendicular to thigh, or slightly angled towards anterior thigh 22–25 gauge (⅝–1 inch)	Insert needle perpendicular to site but angled slightly towards iliac crest 22–25 gauge (½–1 inch)	Insert needle perpendicular to site but angled slightly towards shoulder 22–25 gauge (½–1 inch)

TABLE 5.7 Intramuscular injection sites in children *continued*

	VASTUS LATERALIS (see Fig. 5.16a)	VENTROGLUTEAL (see Fig. 5.16b)	DELTOID (see Fig. 5.17)
Advantages	Large, well-developed muscle that can tolerate larger quantities of fluid (0.5 mL [infant] to 2.0 mL [child]). Easily accessible if child is supine, side-lying or sitting	Free of important nerves and vascular structures. Easily identified by prominent bony landmarks. Thinner layer of subcutaneous tissue than in dorsogluteal site, thus less chance of depositing drug subcutaneously rather than intramuscularly. Can accommodate larger quantities of fluid (0.5 mL [infant] to 2.0 mL [child]). Easily accessible if child is supine, prone or side-lying. Less painful than vastus lateralis	Faster absorption rates than gluteal sites. Easily accessible with minimal removal of clothing. Less pain and fewer local side effects from vaccines compared with vastus lateralis
Disadvantages	Thrombosis of femoral artery from injection in midthigh area. Sciatic nerve damage from long needle injected posteriorly and medially into small extremity. More painful than deltoid or gluteal sites	Health professionals' unfamiliarity with site	Small muscle mass; only limited amounts of drug can be injected (0.5–1.0 mL). Small margins of safety with possible damage to radial nerve and axillary nerve (not shown; lies under deltoid at head of humerus)

*Locations are indicated by asterisks in Figs 5.16 and 5.17. (From Hockenberry et al 2019.)

- The viscosity of the medication to be given.
- The amount and general condition of the muscle mass on the paediatric patient.
- The frequency of the medication.
- The type of medication.
- Factors that may cause contamination.
- The ability of the paediatric patient to be placed or place themselves in a safe position.

(Adapted from Anderson & Herring 2019, p 711.)

Injections must be administered into muscles large enough to accommodate the volume of medication while also avoiding nerves and blood vessels (Anderson & Herring 2019, p 711) (also see Box 5.3).

Box 5.3
General tips in administering IM injections

- Explain what is to be done to the caregiver and seek consent
- Establish how the caregiver can help and what the paediatric patient can do to assist, if able
- In preparing the paediatric patient for an injection the choice of words should be considered. Children may associate 'needle' with punishment. 'Putting the medication under the skin' may be a preferred choice of words
- Because injections are painful, excellent technique is required and appropriate age-related pain reduction measures
- Distract the paediatric patient with conversation or items
  - Give the paediatric patient something to concentrate on – squeezing a hand, counting to 10, humming, etc.
  - Use a cooling agent on the site prior to the injection, for example, a cold compress
- Children are generally unpredictable and even if they appear relaxed, the stress of having an injection may cause them to move. Prepare the paediatric patient with the appropriate holding technique. It is recommended that a second person is available
  - Ventrogluteal – position paediatric patient on side with upper leg flexed and placed in front of lower leg
  - Vastus lateralis – supine, lying on side or sitting
- Allow the skin preparation to dry before inserting the needle
- Grasp the muscle firmly between the thumb and fingers to isolate and stabilise the muscle
- Insert the needle in a dartlike motion at a 90-degree angle unless otherwise contraindicated
- As the needle is inserted avoid the plunger being depressed – wait until the needle is in

Box 5.3
General tips in administering IM injections *continued*

- After administering, remove the needle quickly – dispose of the needle
- Apply pressure to the injection site – apply an adhesive Band-Aid and a smiley face
- Encourage caregivers to hold and cuddle the paediatric patient
- Allow expression of feelings
- Reward paediatric patient

(Adapted from Anderson & Herring 2019 in Hockenberry et al 2019.)

Nursing alert

- The dorsogluteal site (buttocks) is no longer recommended as a site for IM injections of children under 10 years (Brown et al in Anderson & Herring 2019 in Hockenberry et al 2019)
- Aspiration during IM injection is no longer recommended; however, it may still be indicated for injections such as penicillin in larger muscle groups, for example, the ventrogluteal (Anderson & Herring 2019)
- It is recommended to follow organisation policy
- When preparing injection from a glass ampoule always use a filter drawing-up needle to prevent glass aspiration

SUBCUTANEOUS AND INTRADERMAL INJECTIONS

Subcutaneous and intradermal injections are frequently administered to children (Table 5.8).

The different angles for insertion with IM, intradermal and subcutaneous injections are illustrated in Figure 5.17.

Techniques to minimise the pain include:

- Using a 26–30-gauge needle to inject the solution
- Injecting small volumes (≤ 0.5 mL)

TABLE 5.8 Examples of medications via subcutaneous or intradermal

SUBCUTANEOUS INJECTIONS	INTRADERMAL INJECTIONS
Insulin, hormone replacement, allergy desensitisation, vaccines	Tuberculin testing, local anaesthesia, allergy testing

(Anderson & Herring 2019.)

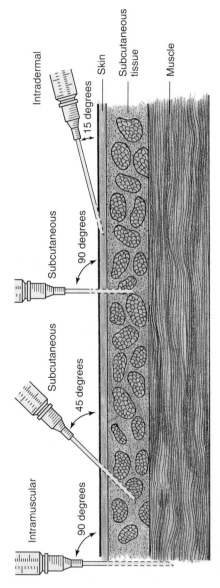

Figure 5.17 Comparison of angles of insertion for intramuscular (90 degrees), subcutaneous (45 degrees) and intradermal (15 degrees) injections. (Crisp et al 2013.)

- The angle of a subcutaneous injection is typically 90 degrees; however, if the paediatric patient has little subcutaneous fat some nurses may consider 45 degrees (this remains controversial).

Subcutaneous injection sites include:
- Anterior abdominal wall (site of choice)
- Anterior aspect of the upper arms
- Anterior aspect of the thigh.

When frequent administration is required (e.g., insulin administration in a patient with diabetes mellitus or daily heparin injections) administration sites should be rotated (Fig. 5.18).

The skill of administering IM, subcutaneous and intradermal injections to a paediatric patient requires an emphasis on the

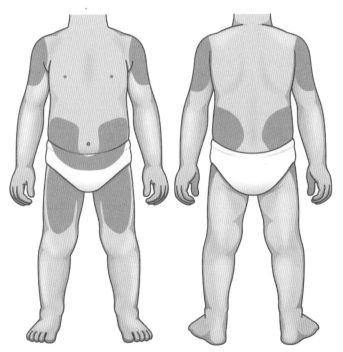

Figure 5.18 Sites for rotating subcutaneous injections. (Source: https://www.kineretrx.com/nomid/using-kineret.)

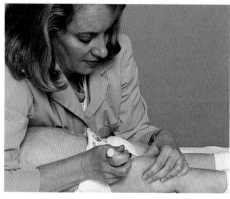

Figure 5.19 Holding a small child for intramuscular injection. Note how the nurse isolates and stabilises the muscle. (Hockenberry et al 2019.)

correct checking of the medication and understanding of site selection, as well as communication, cooperation and appropriate holding/positioning, as seen in Figure 5.19.

To gain further understanding of preparing and administering IM and subcutaneous injections refer to Paediatric skill 7.7 in Chapter 7.

INTRAVENOUS MEDICATIONS

The IV route is common for medication administration and fluid replacement in paediatric patients.

Reasons for a paediatric patient to require IV include:

- Replacement of fluids from diarrhoea/vomiting
- When needing a high serum concentration of a drug
- When the paediatric patient has resistant infections that require parental medications over an extended time
- When needing continuous pain relief
- In emergency treatment.

(Adapted from Anderson & Herring 2019, p 714.)

The nurse needs to consider several factors with IV administration of medications, including:

- The effect is almost instantaneous, and control of side effects is limited

- Most IV medications require specified minimum dilution, rate of flow or both
- Many IV medications must be prepared from a powder solution
- IV medications can be irritating or toxic to tissues outside of the vascular access.
  (Anderson & Herring 2019, p 714.)

If a paediatric patient needs to have an IV medication or IV fluids, the nurse may be required to assist with the set-up in preparation for insertion of an IV cannula and the securing of that site. This will involve preparing the paediatric patient and their caregiver, gathering the equipment, and supporting the paediatric patient and medical officer through the process.

Preparing paediatric patient and caregiver for IV cannula insertion

Assisting with intravenous access

If the paediatric patient does not already have an IV cannula where the medication can be administered, the nurse may be required to assist in the set-up and administration.

Considerations include:

- Education and consent of the caregiver and paediatric patient is a priority
- Preparation for distraction activities is important.
- When a decision is made in terms of access sites, the nurse can apply the appropriate numbing cream with a film over-lay (Fig. 5.20).
- The paediatric patient's age, developmental, cognitive and mobility needs must be considered when choosing a site.
- The older paediatric patient may choose their preferred site.
- A near-infrared imaging device can aid in finding and evaluating vein access.
- Pain relief, mild sedation should be considered as prescribed by the medical officer.
- Some organisations will have a policy in place specifying how many attempts the medical officer can have to insert an IV cannula (e.g., three). The nurse needs to be prepared to speak up if the number of permitted attempts is breached.

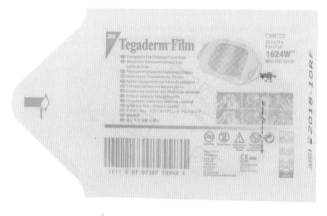

Figure 5.20 Example of numbing cream and film dressing overlay. 3M™ Tegaderm™ Transparent Film Dressing Courtesy of 3M. ©3M 2016. All rights reserved.

Equipment required for insertion of peripheral IV cannula

Thorough preparation for insertion is essential in facilitating a smooth process. When equipment is not on hand, sites can be lost and the trauma for the paediatric patient and caregiver can be enhanced. The decision around the size of the cannula will be determined by the medical officer. The smallest gauge cannula and shortest length appropriate for the paediatric patient's size should be chosen. The gauge should also be sufficient to allow appropriate flow. The nurse should have the selected site dressing, tapes, arm board and bandage ready on hand to secure the cannula after insertion (Fig. 5.21).

During the procedure the nurse will support the medical officer and paediatric patient in the following ways:

- Reassurance to the paediatric patient, caregiver
- Support in securing the arm for insertion – having the required number of persons to assist is important
- Providing distraction techniques
- Having lines primed and ready to hand to the medical officer, or allocating to another nurse
- Securing the site.

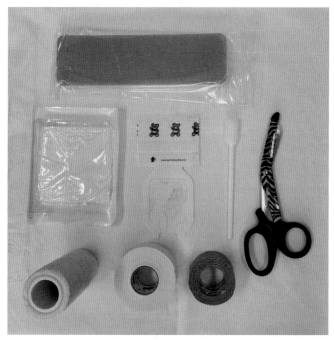

Figure 5.21 Equipment needed for IV insertion.

Maintenance of IV therapy in the paediatric patient can be difficult because of factors such as:
- Vascular trauma from having the cannula inserted
- Vessel size
- Vessel fragility
- Pump pressure
- Activity level of the paediatric patient
- Operator skill
- Insertion technique
- Forceful administration of bolus fluids
- The infusion of irritants or vesicants through a small vessel

(Anderson & Herring 2019, p 723.)

Securement of peripheral intravenous cannula

IV cannulas must be stabilised to allow inspection, prevent dislodgement, and allow administration of medication.

To maintain protection (Fig. 5.22):

- Ensure catheter hub is firmly secured with appropriate paediatric transparent film IV dressing.

Securing a PIVC in the hand

Place splint with foam facing the skin under the hand and wrist. Use pre-prepared splinting board tapes to attach the splinting. Keep the thumb free for patient to use. Ensure that fingers are firmly secured, but not so tight as to cause pressure areas. Ensure that the cannula site can be easily accessed for regular assessment. Use some brown tape to keep extension from moving. Be aware of potential pressure areas when placing this tape.

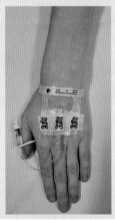

Securing a PIVC in the antecubital fossa

Antecubital fossa cannulas should be used as a last resort. They are appropriate in emergencies where immediate IV access is required for investigations and treatment to commence.

Place the splint with the foam side facing the skin under the elbow. Use two pre-prepared tapes to attach the splinting. Gently apply a third pre-prepared tape across the cannula insertion site. Ensure that the cannula site can be easily accessed for regular assessment.

Figure 5.22 Securing PIVC.

- The dressing should be dated indicating when the cannula was inserted. This should also be documented in the paediatric patient notes.
- Avoid tapes that prevent inspection of site – the site proximal to insertion site should be visible.
- Place securement device.
- Devices applied should be easily managed to allow hourly inspection of the site.
- IV tubing should be secured to prevent infants and children pulling at this.
- Fingers and toes should be left uncovered by dressings to allow inspection for assessment of circulation.
- The thumb should never be immobilised due to risk of contractures.
- An extremity should never be circled with tape as circulation could be compromised.
- Caution in using padded arm boards or splints – they can:
    - restrict access to a site
    - cause contractures
    - be uncomfortable
    - restrict movement.
- Once secure, the site should be easily accessed for inspection.
- The site should be secure to prevent access by the paediatric patient.
- The paediatric patient name band/bracelet should not be on the extremity where the peripheral IV site is located as this could act as a tourniquet and thus impair circulation.

Nursing alert

Opaque covering should be avoided to secure an IV site. The insertion site and extremity distal to the site should be visible to detect infiltration or phlebitis.

Inspection of IV site

When a medication is being administered or fluids are being infused, the cannula site and the associated extremity should be inspected hourly. Documentation of findings is important.

Infiltration is when the medication or non-vesicant fluid goes into the surrounding tissue. This can arise due to the dislodgement of the cannula. If the fluid or medication was vesicant, that is, causing injury to surrounding tissue, this would be referred to as extravasation and further management is required.

The nurse should monitor for signs of dislodgement, infiltration, extravasation or phlebitis (see Table 5.9) by noting:

- Colour
- Warmth
- Movement
- Sensation
- Capillary refill.

It should be noted that the early detection of infiltration on an infant is more difficult because of the amount of subcutaneous fat, the dressing, bandages and taping required for stabilisation of the cannula (Anderson & Herring 2019, p 723).

It should be noted that there are three types of phlebitis:

- Mechanical – caused by rapid infusion rate and manipulation of the IV
- Chemical – caused by medication
- Bacterial – caused by staphylococcal infection.

If a nurse notices signs of dislodgement, infiltration, extravasation or phlebitis the action should be:

- Stop the infusion
- Elevate the extremity
- Notify a doctor
- Initiate management as ordered
- Remove cannula.

(Anderson & Herring 2019, p 723.)

TABLE 5.9 Signs of dislodgement, infiltration, extravasation and phlebitis

DISLODGEMENT	INFILTRATION	EXTRAVASATION	PHLEBITIS
Bandage/film dressing wet	Swelling Cool to touch Complaints of discomfort	Erythema Pain Oedema Blanching Streaking along the vein Darkened area at the insertion site	Redness at site Pain at site may or may not be present

Nursing alert

The most effective way to prevent infection at the IV site is to adhere to the five moments of hand hygiene, wear gloves on insertion and inspect the site regularly, ensuring that visibility is clear. Education to the patient and caregiver about preventing infection and monitoring signs is important (Hockenberry et al 2019, p 723; Hand Hygiene Australia 2023).

General tips on speaking up

A nurse may be assisting with the insertion of an IV cannula and notices a breach in infection control. For example, the appropriately qualified nurse:

- Fails to cleanse the cannula site with the appropriate cleansing swab
- Cleanses the site then palpates the insertion site with a non-gloved finger
- Cleanses the site then cuts the tip of the glove off to expose their finger to palpate the site

All of these are examples of practices which can pose a risk of infection. The nurse has a responsibility to speak up and point out that infection control has been breached.

Preparing IV medications

As covered in this guide already, the preparation of any medication being delivered to the paediatric patient requires two people. In addition to what has already been covered in medication administration, special considerations for IV infusion include:

- A clear understanding of the amount of medication to be administered. The nurse should use the injectables guidelines for checking of:
  - drug name
  - actions
  - interactions
  - recommended dose per weight
  - side effects
  - duration that the drug can be administered over
  - what compatible fluid the drug can be diluted with and if the drug is compatible with the fluid that is running and with any other medications the paediatric patient may be prescribed.

- The minimum dilution must be checked.
- Whether paediatric patient is on a fluid restriction.
- The completion of additive labels.
  (Adapted from Hockenberry et al 2019, p 714.)

Key tips in preparing IV medications

When preparing IV medications the nurse should have a second qualified person checking from preparation to administration. The nurse should adhere to the six rights and checks, as explained previously. The correct use of PPE is important.

All equipment should be on hand, including:
- Medication chart
- Complete order
- Medication
- Appropriate injectable guidelines for paediatrics
- Syringe
- Appropriate drawing-up needles
- IV access devices
- Alcohol swabs
- Solution for drawing up
- Solution for infusing
- Appropriate IV needleless tubing
- Infusion pump
- Burettes.

When preparing IV medications, many of the medications come in a powder solution (Fig. 5.23). It is very important to follow the manufacturer's instructions or injectable guidelines regarding how much solution to add to the vial. The final volume, which will dictate dose, for example, in mg/mL, will have taken the powder volume into consideration.

To gain further understanding of preparing IV injections refer to Paediatric skill 7.2 in Chapter 7.

Additive labels

When nurses are preparing any IV medication they must complete an additive label (Fig. 5.24), which will be secured to the device in which the medication is being administered; for example, a syringe on a syringe driver (Fig. 5.25), or a burette attached to an infusion line and pump (Fig. 5.26).

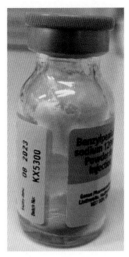

Figure 5.23 Powder for reconstitution.

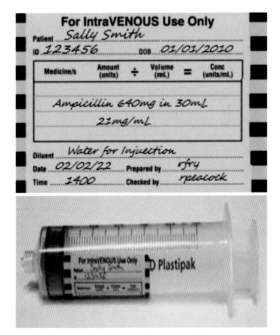

Figure 5.24 Medication label for a syringe driver.

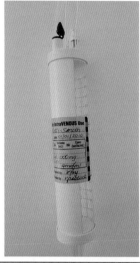

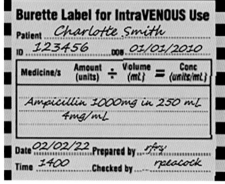

Burette Label for IntraVENOUS Use

Patient .... *Charlotte Smith* ....

ID .... *123456* .... DOB *01/01/2010* ....

Medicine/s	Amount (units)	÷	Volume (ml)	=	Conc (units/ml)
Ampicillin 1000mg in 250 mL					
4mg/mL					

Date *02/02/22* Prepared by *sfry*

Time *1400* Checked by *peacock*

Figure 5.25 Medication label for a burette.

Key points with additive labels

- The label should be completed by the person preparing the medication and checked and signed by the second person
- The label must be affixed to the front of the burette, IV bag or syringe if going via an infusion pump
- If attached to an IV bag, the manufacturer's labelling of product name, batch, expiry date must remain clearly visible
- The fluid levels in the bag must remain clearly visible

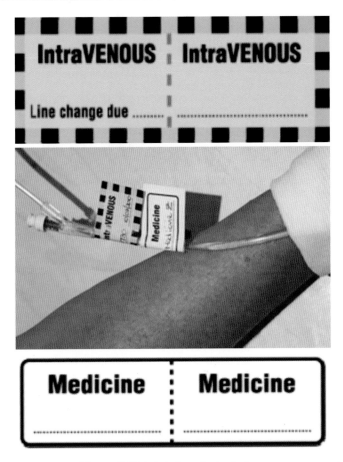

Figure 5.26 Labels for adhering to lines.

- The label should include:
  - patient name, UR number, DOB
  - generic name of medication and dose
  - solution the medication is prepared in
  - concentration and dilution written in dose per mL
  - signatures of person preparing and person checking
  - time and date being administered.

Also see Box 5.4.

Box 5.4
General tips in administering IV injections

- Explain what is to be done to the caregiver and seek consent
- Establish how the caregiver can help and what the paediatric patient can do to assist if able
- In preparing the paediatric patient for an IV injection – the choice of words should be considered
- If the drug is to be administered over a period of time, tell the paediatric patient and caregiver the duration
- Educate the paediatric patient and caregiver not to touch any settings on the pumps but to call for the nurse if the alarms are on
- Because some IV injections can be painful, flucloxacillin for example, provide the paediatric patient with an age-appropriate distraction
- Before administering:
  - undertake all the appropriate checks and rights as for any medication
  - check the IV cannulation site for patency
  - check for signs of dislodgement, infiltration, extravasation, phlebitis
  - if putting the medication into a burette:
    ○ clean the top access bung
    ○ put the required solution into the burette, checking compatibility with the drug
    ○ inject the pre-prepared drug into the burette with a follow through of a small amount of normal saline at the bung site so that no drug remains in the bung
      - set the infusion pump
- Reward paediatric patient with something that the caregiver is agreeable to

Nursing alert

Before administering IV medications
- Have second person checking
- Undertake six rights for medication administration and checks
- Check IV site for patency, which includes flushing easily without resistance or brisk blood return
- If there is resistance do not proceed – the integrity of the access needs to be reviewed
- Check for signs of infiltration or phlebitis
- Do not administer IV medications in the same line as blood products
- Give one medication at a time
- Check the correct dilution and safe volume for infants and children
- Check organisation policy re use of infusion pump or driver
- Check IV site is secure and easily accessible for site inspection

Pushing an IV medication

Pushing IV medications (administering medications intravenously using a syringe rather than an infusion) to a paediatric patient warrants caution. It is important that the decision to do so is in line with recommendations as per the drug manufacturer's instructions and/or *The Australian Injectable Drugs Handbook*.

If pushing a medication, then the following must be adhered to:

- the drug is diluted with the recommended volume and type of solution
- the volume is pushed over the recommended time duration
- the drug is flushed following the push with the required volume of recommended compatible solution (usually 0.9% saline)
- the paediatric patient can tolerate the push considering their size, vein, discomfort
- the site is inspected prior to the push for any signs of infiltration, extravasation or phlebitis.

Infusions

In most instances IV medications to children are administered via an infusion pump.

A variety of infusion pumps (Figs 5.27 & 5.28) are available and are used in nearly all paediatric infusions to administer medications with accuracy and to minimise possible overloading of the circulation with too much fluid.

The nurse should be familiar with the infusion pump including:

- How to set it up.
- How to problem solve.
- How to clean.
- How to use smart pump technology, for example, *guard rails*. Smart infusion pump technology provides built-in features that can alert the nurse when the pump settings are outside programmed parameters, thereby reducing infusion errors. The smart pump technology is programmed with dose and infusion rate information for commonly used medications. It can recognise drug information in its database, check dosing, calculate infusions, monitor line pressure and report errors back to nursing. Guard rails should be used according to the medication being administered, the volume to infuse and the rate.

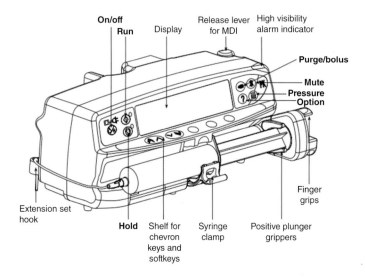

On/off
Run
Display
Release lever for MDI
High visibility alarm indicator
Purge/bolus
Mute
Pressure
Option
Finger grips
Extension set hook
Hold
Shelf for chevron keys and softkeys
Syringe clamp
Positive plunger grippers

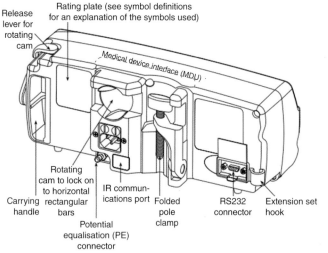

Release lever for rotating cam
Rating plate (see symbol definitions for an explanation of the symbols used)
Medical device interface (MDI)
Rotating cam to lock on to horizontal rectangular bars
Carrying handle
IR communications port
Potential equalisation (PE) connector
Folded pole clamp
RS232 connector
Extension set hook

Figure 5.27 Features of an infusion pump. Courtesy and © Becton, Dickinson and Company.

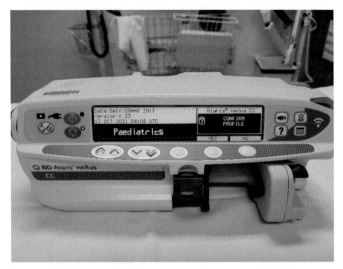

Figure 5.28 Image of an infusion pump. Courtesy and © Becton, Dickinson and Company.

When using infusion pumps the nurse needs to:
- Calculate the amount to be infused in a given length of time
- Set the infusion rate
- Monitor the infusion hourly to ensure:
  - the desired rate is maintained
  - the integrity of the system remains intact
  - the site remains intact, free of infiltration signs and phlebitis
  - the infusion does not stop
- Caregivers should be advised that when pumps are used, nurses are required to check the pump and the infusion site and associated limbs hourly, and should document this
- Education to caregivers about the risk of infiltration is important
- Caregivers should also be advised not to tamper with the pump in any way, including turning it off
- Nurses should avoid separating the access line to the pump for the purposes of toileting and showering.
  (Adapted from Hockenberry et al 2019, p 714.)

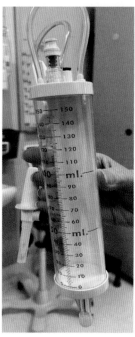

Figure 5.29 A burette. Courtesy and © Becton, Dickinson and Company

Burettes

Burettes (Fig. 5.29) are used for administering IV fluid and for some IV medications to the paediatric patient. Burettes allow the nurse to ensure they administer the correct volume of fluid over a specified time.

> To gain further understanding of preparing and administering IV medications by a syringe driver refer to Paediatric skill 7.2 in Chapter 7.

Removal of intravenous cannulas

Removal of an IV cannula can be anxiety-provoking for a paediatric patient. The nurse needs to provide an explanation of the process. The paediatric patient may want to help in taking off the tapes. The process for removal includes:

- Donning PPE
- Having the required equipment – a swap and film dressing

- Turning off the pumps to cease IV flow
- Removing the tape and film – avoid using scissors
- Pulling the cannula out in the opposite direction of insertion
- Placing the dressing over the site
- Applying gentle compression
- Inspecting the cannula tip to ensure it is intact
- Discarding the cannula and used dressings in appropriate waste container
- Documenting the removal and date
- Monitoring the paediatric patient after the removal
- Rewarding the paediatric patient with something that the caregiver is agreeable to.

CENTRAL VENOUS ACCESS DEVICES

PICC lines

A peripherally inserted central catheter (PICC) is inserted into the brachial vein in the arm and the catheter travels down the superior vena cava into the cavo-atrial junction of the heart (Fig. 5.30).

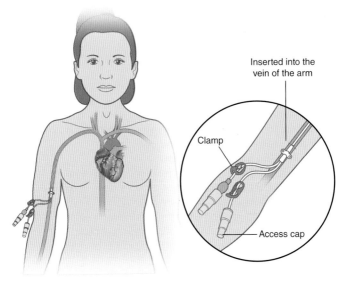

Figure 5.30 Peripherally inserted central catheter (PICC).

Common complications include:
- Blockage
- Infection.

Medical officers may choose to use a central line instead of a regular IV line because:
- It can stay in longer (up to a year or even more)
- It makes it easier to draw blood samples
- The patient can receive large amounts of fluids or medicine (e.g., chemotherapy).

The care, management and delivery of fluids and medication via these devices is similar to the delivery via IV catheter.

The risk of severe infection increases significantly for patients with a PICC due to the close proximity of the catheter to the heart. Any infection will progress quickly, and patients can rapidly become septic. Due care and the highest level of infection prevention must be taken.

RECTALLY ADMINISTERED MEDICATIONS

The administration of rectal medication is not uncommon in the paediatric patient. For example, paracetamol via suppository is ideal for the infant or small paediatric patient who is febrile, vomiting or refusing oral paracetamol.

The advantage is that there is no need to coax the paediatric patient to swallow unpleasant medication.

The absorption by the rectal mucosa is dependent on:
- Gut motility
- The amount of time the drug remains in the rectum
- The amount of stool present at the time of administration.
  To administer:
- Adhere to the usual checking requirements, the six rights of medication administration and consent
- Apply PPE – non-sterile gloves
- Remove the plastic covering from the suppository
- Have the paediatric patient lie on their side with top leg flexed
- Consider distraction strategies
- Insert with pointy end first (Fig. 5.31)
- Gently push in with finger beyond the sphincter
- Hold the buttocks together until urge to expel has passed
- Doff PPE
- Document and monitor effects
- Educate the paediatric patient and caregiver of what to expect.

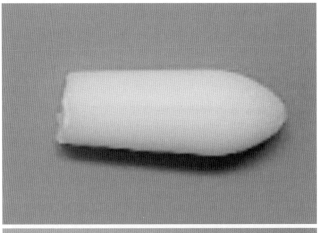

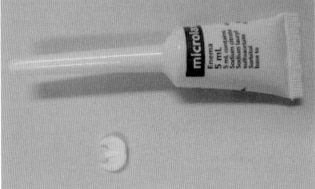

Figure 5.31 Rectal suppository showing pointed end and enema showing pointed end.

To gain further understanding of preparing and administering rectal medication refer to Paediatric skill 7.4 in Chapter 7.

NEBULISED MEDICATIONS

This is an effective method to distribute medication directly to the airways. These medications are suspended particulates, which are inhaled to reach the smaller airways. Medications include bronchodilators, steroids and antibiotics.

Considerations:
- Age of paediatric patient
- Use of oxygen versus air
- Other devices in use that may alter the administration of the correct dose
- Dilution of medications (if required).

  Equipment (Fig. 5.32):
- Appropriate size nebuliser mask and tubing
- Medication, normal saline (if required) for dilution.

Inhaler

Metered dose inhalers (MDI) should be used in conjunction with spacers and, for younger children, masks to ensure effective delivery of medication to the airways.

The use of the spacer, with or without a mask, is to ensure that the metered dose of medication is delivered without reliance on the coordination of breathing by the paediatric patient.

Considerations:
- Age of paediatric patient
- Use of procedural holding with paediatric patient (see Holding/restraint in Ch 4)
- Positioning of paediatric patient to ensure dosage administration

  Equipment:
- MDI
- Spacer/mask (Fig. 5.33)
- Medication

  Method:
1. Shake medication and put in opposite end of spacer to mouthpiece/mask, prime the chamber with multiple puffs (this will help reduce static build-up inside of chamber)
2. Place spacer mouthpiece in mouth, or place mask on paediatric patient's face, ensuring good seal around nose and mouth
3. After exhale of breath, depress medication, the paediatric patient then breathes in the medication; repeat breathing four times
4. Continue from step 1 for further doses.

The following website is a useful resource for information in relation to the use and care of MDIs and spacers: Asthma Australia (https://asthma.org.au/).

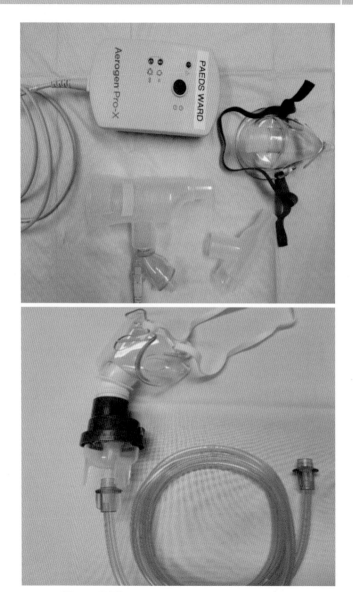

Figure 5.32 Equipment for nebulised medications.

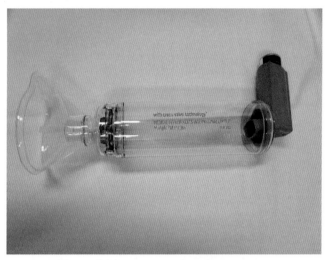

Figure 5.33 Spacer for metered dose inhaler.

To gain further understanding of preparing and administering MDI refer to Paediatric skill 7.5 in Chapter 7.

INTRANASALLY ADMINISTERED MEDICATIONS

Intranasally administered medications are delivered via the highly vascularised nasal mucosa with the use of a mucosal atomisation device (MAD). Several medications are delivered by this route for a variety of conditions, from bronchodilators to sedatives.

The atomiser (Fig. 5.34) is inserted into the nostrils and the medication delivered in even doses to both sides.

MEDICATIONS ADMINISTERED VIA A NASOGASTRIC TUBE

Medications given via the nasogastric route require caution. The correct placement of the tube is paramount.

Prior to administering any medication via this route, the nurse should adhere strictly to the organisation policy including insertion, checking of location and medications appropriate for administration.

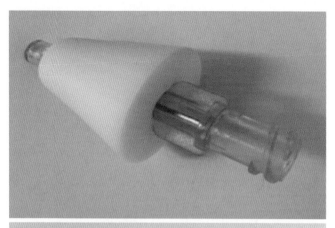

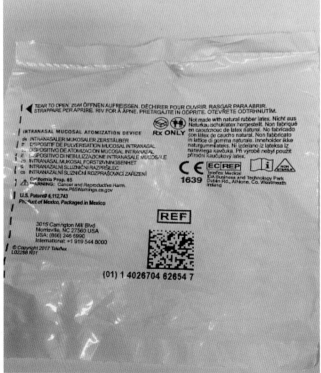

Figure 5.34 Mucosal atomisation device.

The insertion of a nasogastric tube (NGT) is performed by an experienced nurse.

To gain further understanding of administration via NGT, refer to Paediatric skill 7.1 in Chapter 7.

ADMINISTERING MEDICATIONS VIA A PEG

Percutaneous endoscopic gastrostomy (PEG) is a tube inserted directly into the stomach.

The tube is surgically inserted through the abdominal wall, midway at the greater curvature of the stomach; the stomach is then secured to the peritoneum, creating a stoma. The stoma is then fixed with a device called a MIC-KEY or Bard button, a silicon device that protrudes slightly from the skin, which can be submerged in water and has a one-way valve (Fig. 5.35).

Specialised equipment is used to access these devices, which require nursing knowledge of how to use them. Care is necessary when using these devices for medication administration, ensuring that they do not become clogged due to the viscosity or by sediments of the medication.

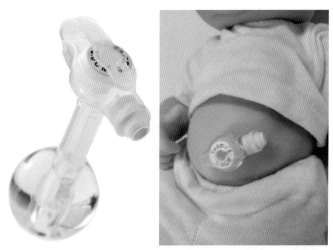

Figure 5.35 MIC-KEY.

Nursing considerations:
- Hand hygiene and gloves
- PEG attachment
- Medication in liquid form, elixir or crushed and dissolved
- Syringes
- Water to flush
- Knowledge of PEG and use.

(Adapted from Anderson & Herring 2019.)

INTRAOSSEOUS ADMINISTRATION OF MEDICATION

Intraosseous (IO) access is used in emergency situations and is an effective route for fluid resuscitation, drug delivery and laboratory evaluation that may be used in all age groups. Insertion of an IO requires a specific drill and the appropriate size needles contained within a preparation kit (Fig. 5.36).

The IO space functions as a non-collapsible vein. To view the insertion of an IO, refer to the following guidelines and YouTube presentation:

- The Royal Children's Hospital Melbourne, Clinical Practice Guidelines: Intraosseous access (https://www.rch.org.au/clinicalguide/guideline_index/Intraosseous_access/)

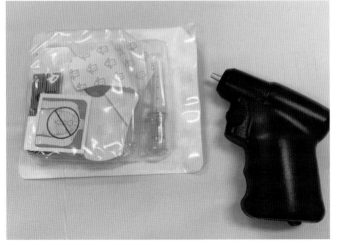

Figure 5.36 Intraosseous drill and kit.

- YouTube: Arrow® EZ-IO® Infant Child Needle Selection
  and Insertion Technique Animation Video (https://www.
  youtube.com/watch?v=mpnroZi8t0A.)
  Once an IO is inserted, nursing care includes:
- Hourly neurovascular observations
- Observing for the following complications:
  - discolouration of limb
  - swelling
  - increased pain
  - altered sensation in limb
  - temperature changes.

The care, management and delivery of fluids and medication
via an IO is similar to the delivery via IV catheter.

The risk of infection increases significantly for patients with an
IO, as the device goes directly into the bone marrow. Any infection
will progress quickly, and patients can rapidly become septic. Due
care and the highest level of infection prevention must be taken.

Specialised/ high-risk paediatric medication

Pauline Davies, Rinnah Peacock, Kerry Reid-Searl

High-risk medicines (HRMs) are medications that have an increased risk of causing significant patient harm or death if they are misused or used in error (Australian Commission on Safety and Quality in Health Care 2022).

Specialised and high-risk medications will require extra knowledge, training and competencies to handle and safely administer these medications. Check local health service policies, guidelines and pharmacy for skills and competencies required for the use, handling and administration of these medications.

Immunisations

Immunisations are in accordance with the Australian National Immunisation Program Schedule. All other countries need to follow their own organisation's/government's recommendations for immunisation programs.

Nurses need to be aware of the schedules and the practices of each organisation regarding immunisation and keep abreast of the most up-to-date information and changes in schedules. Children who have not received immunisations due to illnesses, treatments or beliefs are eligible to have the immunisations in a catch-up format.

Note: in Australia, the Aboriginal and Torres Strait Islander populations have a different immunisation schedule.

For further information, refer to the *Australian Immunisation Handbook* (Australian Government, Department of Health and Aged Care 2018 [https://immunisationhandbook.health.gov.au/]).

Checks when administering immunisations:

- Does the nurse have vaccination accreditation or has an order been written by the doctor?
- Is there a medication order or has the accredited vaccination nurse completed appropriate paperwork and checked immunisation schedule?
- Has consent been obtained?
- Has the paediatric patient had a previous reaction, or allergies to the ingredients in some immunisations?
- Have the six checks occurred with an age and schedule check as well?
- Has there been sufficient time between vaccines?
- Has the vaccine been kept in a vaccine fridge with no cold chain breach?
- Has there been documentation of vaccine, including injection site and serial number of vaccines to appropriate authorities to ensure registration of immunisation?

Chemotherapy

Additional qualifications and chemotherapy competency are required for the administration of chemotherapy in paediatrics. The dosing of chemotherapy is carried out by a Paediatric Oncologist, following specific treatment protocols.

Due to the working of chemotherapy agents, most patients receiving chemotherapy will be immunocompromised and therefore if presenting unwell will need immediate treatment in conjunction with protective isolation as they are at high risk of sepsis. Known as febrile neutropenia or non-neutropenia the patient will require antibiotics according to local hospital flow charts, protocols and policies.

Immediate treatment includes:

- Central venous access device (CVAD), totally implantable venous access device (TIVAD) or portacath (POC) access and collection of bloods

- Intravenous antibiotics as charted to be administered within 1 hour of presentation to hospital.

Chemotherapy medication is administered by registered nurses (RNs) who have completed oncology administration competency and training in side effects of a vesicant and non-vesicant drug and precautions. The same is required for the appropriately qualified nurse or pharmacist, double-checking the chemotherapy agent being administered.

Nursing considerations:
- CVAD (TIVAD or POC) qualifications
- Chemotherapy competent
- Appropriate personal protective equipment (PPE) and preparation for cytotoxic spills and extravasation
- Knowledge of procedures and guidelines.

Note: there are other conditions and diseases that use chemotherapy agents in their treatment; for example, juvenile idiopathic arthritis (JIA) and irritable bowel disease (IBD) of which the appropriately qualified nurse will need to be cyctoxic aware.

Insulin

Insulin is a drug used to correct the body's glucose levels, where the body has been unable to maintain its own glucose levels by producing insulin in the pancreas. Natural insulin is required to convert the food into glucose that the body will use as energy.

Insulin comes in the form of short/immediate-acting and long/intermediate-acting; these are both given by subcutaneous injection or insulin pump.

The chronic condition where the body has little to no insulin is diabetes mellitus (DM).
- Type 1 DM – is an autoimmune condition in which the immune system attacks the pancreatic cells that produce insulin; there is no known cause or cure.
- Type 2 DM – is when the body becomes resistant to insulin, causing the pancreas to produce less insulin.

Diabetes is a serious complex condition that can affect the entire body; too high levels of glucose in the bloodstream can cause short- and long-term health complications.
- Diabetes ketoacidosis (DKA) is the absence of insulin, causing the body to resort to breaking down fat cells in the body, resulting in fatty acids, which are converted by the liver into

ketones, with the excess eliminated through urine and lungs. Ketones in the bloodstream cause changes in the serum pH, producing ketoacidosis.

The ketoacidosis needs to be treated immediately with a combination of insulin and fluid therapy in conjunction with the correction of electrolyte imbalances.

Refer to the state guidelines for treatment.

Nursing considerations:

- IVC site care
- Fluid balance and fluids
- Bloods, BGL, blood gases
- Education from a multidisciplinary team
- Knowledge of insulin administration and action
- Carbohydrate counting
- Hypoglycaemic management
- Recognition of DKA signs, symptoms and treatment.

The treatment and management of diabetes requires a multidisciplinary and holistic approach, as a diagnosis not only affects the whole of the paediatric patient's life but also the lives of their family. Diabetes Australia is a valuable resource for children and families with diabetes (see website: https://www.diabetesaustralia.com.au/).

REACTIVE AIRWAYS DISEASE

Reactive airways disease is a reaction of the airways to an irritant that causes a chronic inflammatory response of the airway, often referred to as asthma or preschool wheeze. The result of this is tightening of the chest, breathlessness, wheezing and cough. This can be treated with bronchodilators and steroids.

Salbutamol, ipratropium, dexamethasone, prednisolone and magnesium are just some of the medications used in the treatment of reactive airways disease. The administration of these medications varies but have been covered within this book. Please refer to local guidelines for treatment.

Nursing considerations:

- Education of paediatric patient and caregiver
- Use of metered dose inhalers (MDIs) and nebulisers
- Auscultation practices
- Knowledge of the disease process of reactive airways disease
- Use of vasodilators and steroids.

Medications in emergency: resuscitation

The administration of medication to the paediatric patient in resuscitation is performed by paediatric advanced life support qualified nurses. Guidelines will dictate which medications nurses can administer.

Every state of Australia will have specific guidelines for nurses to follow. In Queensland, resources such as the Children's Resuscitation Emergency Drug Dosage (CREDD) have been developed for all types of emergencies. CREDD includes different weights of the paediatric patient and all the calculations for medications according to that weight as well as sizing of equipment that may be required in an emergency. Figure 6.1 shows CREDD and Figure 6.2 highlights the selected drug dosages for a paediatric patient weighing 10 kg.

During an emergency the caregiver may be present. Nursing care will require them to be kept up-to-date of the situation and they may provide information as to the incident or family and medical history. This can be a highly emotive time for the caregiver/s.

Once the primary assessment has been completed and the paediatric patient is stable, a secondary survey should be completed with a complete head-to-toe assessment. This is a time to establish a rapport with the paediatric patient and their significant other/caregiver. Pain management and maintenance of body temperature should be included.

Special considerations

INFECTION CONTROL

Hand hygiene is an absolute requirement in all elements of preparing and administering medication. The five moments of hand hygiene should be in place (Fig. 6.3; Hand Hygiene Australia 2023). Additionally, nurses may be required to use PPE. As such, every nurse should adhere to the policy and procedures around PPE when administering medications (see Table 6.1 for a guide).

- Oral administration – do not touch medication with your hands; dispense directly from the packaging into a medication cup or into an oral syringe
- IV/IM/SC administration – wear gloves when preparing medication
- Special precautions apply for administering chemotherapy medications.

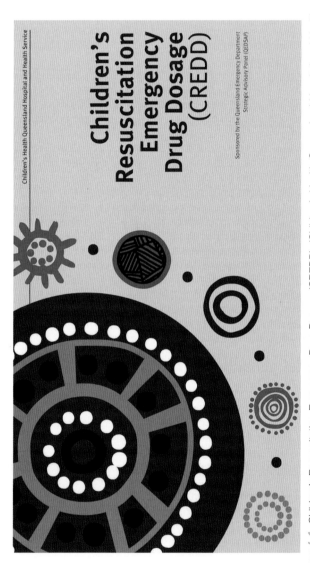

Figure 6.1 Children's Resuscitation Emergency Drug Dosage (CREDD). (Children's Health Queensland Hospital and Health Service 2021. [https://www.childrens.health.qld.gov.au/for-health-professionals/queensland-paediatric-emergency-care-qpec/emergency-medicine-guides.].)

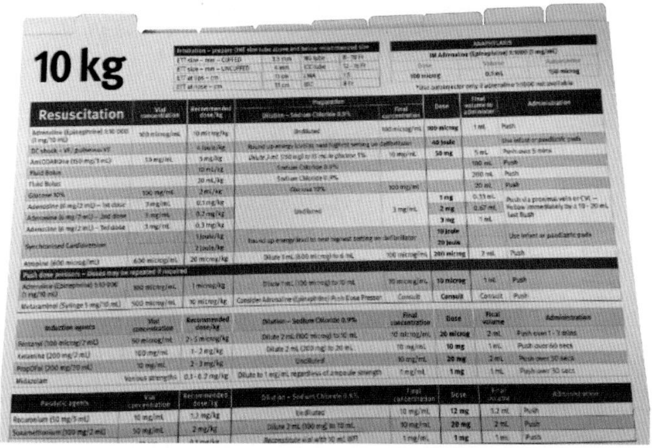

Figure 6.2 Selected drug dosages for a 10-kg paediatric patient.
(Children's Health Queensland Hospital and Health Service 2023 Paediatric
resuscitation tools, Queensland Paediatric Emergency Care [https://www.
childrens.health.qld.gov.au/for-health-professionals/queensland-paediatric-
emergency-care-qpec/queensland-paediatric-resuscitation-tools#tab-
6ff1bb73468033104a2.].)

Being mindful of infection control requirements (e.g., what
can and cannot be removed from isolation rooms) will assist in
the process of medication preparation and administration. The
local organisation's infection control policies will outline PPE
requirements for specific conditions. PPE can create barriers in
communication, as well as fear and anxiety for paediatric
patients. This makes it even more important that nurses implement some of the previously mentioned distraction and communication techniques to gain the paediatric patient's cooperation
for medication administration (Table 6.2).

Nursing alert

The risk of nurses being contaminated with spit and vomit by
children/infants who may be non-compliant, not able to understand,
upset or dislike the taste of a medication is very high. Full PPE
should be worn by the nurse including face mask and goggles.

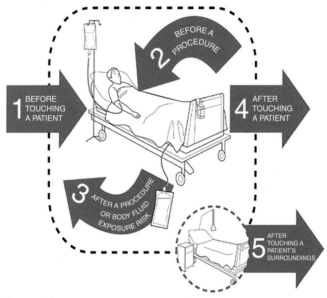

Figure 6.3 Five moments for hand hygiene. (Source: Based on 'My 5 Moments for Hand Hygiene' © World Health Organization 2009. All rights reserved.)

TABLE 6.1 Personal protective equipment (PPE) for medication preparation and administration

PPE	ORAL	IV	SC	PR	NGT	PICC	INTRANASAL
Gloves non-sterile	✓	✓	✓	✓	✓	✓	✓
Gloves sterile							
Apron							
Mask	✓						✓

IV: intravenous; NGT: nasogastric tube; PICC: peripherally inserted central catheter; PR: per rectum; SC: subcutaneous.

TABLE 6.2 Infection control precautions and personal protective equipment (PPE) requirements

PRECAUTIONS	PPE REQUIREMENTS	EXAMPLES OF CONDITIONS
Contact precautions	Glove White gown	MRSA

Guidelines

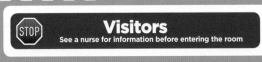

Visitors

STOP See a nurse for information before entering the room

For all staff

Contact Precautions

in addition to Standard Precautions

Before entering room

1 Perform hand hygiene

2 Put on gown or apron

3 Put on gloves

On leaving room

1 Dispose of gloves

2 Perform hand hygiene

3 Dispose of gown or apron

4 Perform hand hygiene

Standard Precautions

And **always** follow these **standard precautions**

- Perform hand hygiene before and after every patient contact
- Use PPE when risk of body fluid exposure

- Use and dispose of sharps safely
- Perform routine environmental cleaning
- Clean and reprocess shared patient equipment

- Follow respiratory hygiene and cough etiquette
- Use aseptic technique
- Handle and dispose of waste and used linen safely

AUSTRALIAN COMMISSION
ON SAFETY AND QUALITY IN HEALTH CARE

Reproduced with permission from *Infection Prevention and Control Poster - Contact precautions poster*, developed by the Australian Commission on Safety and Quality in Health Care (ACSQHC). ACSQHC: Sydney 2023.

Continued

TABLE 6.2 Infection control precautions and personal protective equipment (PPE) requirements *continued*

PRECAUTIONS	PPE REQUIREMENTS	EXAMPLES OF CONDITIONS
Droplet precautions	Gloves Non-pervious gown Mask (surgical) Goggles	RSV

Guidelines

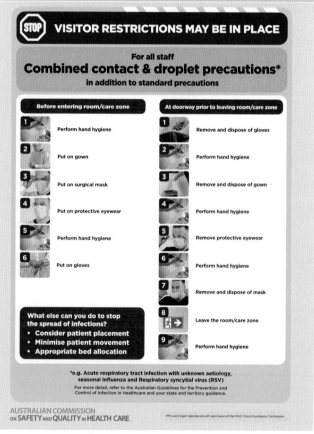

Reproduced with permission from *Infection Prevention and Control Poster - Combined contact and droplet precautions,* developed by the Australian Commission on Safety and Quality in Health Care (ACSQHC). ACSQHC: Sydney 2023.

TABLE 6.2 Infection control precautions and personal protective equipment (PPE) requirements *continued*

PRECAUTIONS	PPE REQUIREMENTS	EXAMPLES OF CONDITIONS
Airborne precautions	Gloves Non-pervious gown Mask (N95, P2) Goggles	Chickenpox COVID-19

Guidelines

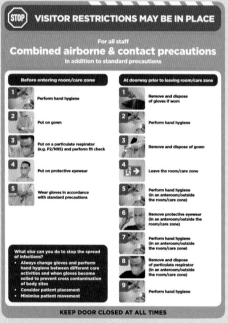

| Cytotoxic precautions (if paediatric patient has had chemotherapy agent in last 7 days) | Purple gloves
Purple gown
If required,
goggles and mask | |

Reproduced with permission from *Infection Prevention and Control Poster - Combined airborne and contact precautions,* developed by the Australian Commission on Safety and Quality in Health Care (ACSQHC). ACSQHC: Sydney 2023.

Interpretation of clinical assessment tools and paediatric medication

CEWT (CHILDREN'S EARLY WARNING TOOL)

See Figure 6.4. Medication that can affect CEWT observations include:

Increase heart rate	Ventolin Decongestants Cold medications ADHD medications
Decrease heart rate	Heart and blood pressure medications Medicines used for depression/ anxiety
Increas blood pressure	NSAIDs (ibuprofen)
Decrease blood pressure	Blood pressure medications

PAIN ASSESSMENT TOOLS

Paediatric nurses play a pivotal role in the managing, preventing and treatment of pain in children, with research showing that untreated acute pain can lead to lifelong chronic pain. It is essential for the paediatric nurse to use the assessment tools (see later in this section), knowledge of developmental ages of children and techniques to assess a paediatric patient in pain.

Children of all ages will experience pain on many different levels, from procedural pain, postoperative pain, headaches, abdominal pain, to chronic conditions and the pain associated with these. Considerations should be made for cultural beliefs, syndromes, diseases, mental capacity and age of paediatric patient, as these will all affect the assessment and treatment of pain.

The complexity of pain experienced by children requires a multidimensional and holistic approach to the management and treatment of pain. Management can consist of pharmacological and non-pharmacological treatments, and can include distraction, heat/cold packs, family assistance, physiotherapy, counsellor, paracetamol, sucrose, ibuprofen and opioids. Please refer to

(Affix identification label here)

URN:

Family name:

Given name(s):

Address:

Date of birth:

Sex: ☐ M ☐ F ☐ I

<1 YEAR

⚠ **Complete Pain Score** (page 4)

CEWT Score Legend

0	Score 0
1	Score 1
2	Score 2
3	Score 3
4	Score 4
E	Emergency Call

Initiate EMERGENCY CALL immediately if any of the following:
- Airway threat
- Apnoea
- Seizure
- Bleeding (major)
- Sedation Score of 3
- Any observation in the purple area (**E**)
- You are worried about the patient

Escalation and Observation Plan (for tertiary and secondary facilities)

For authorised changes to the response for patients with scores ≥8 or E, refer to the MET-MEO (Modified Escalation and Observation plan) on page 1.

CEWT score	Clinical status		Required actions
0	Stable or improving	No concern, and score same or lower	• 8th hourly observations (minimum), unless otherwise authorised by SMO and details documented in patient's medical notes for long stay patients
1–3	Deteriorating	Concern patient is worse or not improving	• 1 hourly observations unless otherwise authorised by SMO and details documented in patient's medical notes for long stay patients
		New contributing vital sign(s)	• Notify Team Leader
		Score higher than last score	• Nurse escort for transfers within facility
	Stable or improving	None of the 3 deteriorating factors above	• 4th hourly observations (minimum), unless otherwise authorised by SMO and details documented in patient's medical notes
4–5	Deteriorating	Concern patient is worse or not improving	• 1 hourly observations
		New contributing vital sign(s)	• Notify Team Leader
			• Notify RMO to review within 30 minutes
			• Nurse escorts for transfers within facility
		Score higher than last score	• If no review after 30 minutes, call Registrar
	Stable or improving	None of the 3 deteriorating factors above	• 2nd hourly observations (minimum), unless otherwise authorised by SMO and details documented in patient's medical notes
6–7	Deteriorating	Concern patient is worse or not improving	• ½ hourly observations
		New contributing vital sign(s)	• Notify Team Leader
			• Notify Registrar to review within 30 minutes
			• Nurse escorts for transfers within facility
		Score higher than last score	• If no review after 30 minutes, call a MET or escalate to SMO
	Stable or improving	None of the 3 deteriorating factors above	• 1 hourly observations (minimum), unless otherwise authorised by SMO and details documented in patient's medical notes
≥8 or E	Deteriorating	Concern patient is worse or not improving	• Initiate MET call (unless ARP suggests alternative non-MET escalation)
		New contributing vital sign(s)	• 10 minutely observations (unless on terminal care pathway)
			• Registrar to ensure SMO is notified
		Score higher than last score	• Registrar and Nurse escort for transfers within facility

Could it be sepsis?

Commence the Paediatric Sepsis Pathway if the patient has a known or signs of suspected infection plus any of the following:

- Looks sick or toxic
- Altered behaviour or reduced level of consciousness
- Re-presentation with same illness
- Sepsis admission within the last 30 days
- Parental and/or clinician concern
- Age younger than 3 months
- Immunocompromised
- Aboriginal or Torres Strait Islander person

*For oncology patients refer to 'Management of suspected neutropenic sepsis' pathway

Features of severe illness:

- Severe respiratory distress or tachypnoea or apnoea (CEWT Respiratory Score 3)
- Altered AVPU
- Poor skin perfusion or cold extremities
- Hypotension (CEWT Systolic Blood Pressure 2 or more)
- Severe tachycardia (CEWT Heart Rate 3)

Laboratory features of severe illness (if known):

- Lactate >2 mmol/L
- Elevated creatinine
- Low platelets
- Elevated INR or bilirubin
- Elevated CRP

Notification Legend

Document the letter(s) in the *Notification* row on page 2 in appropriate time column.

| N | Nil Required | RMO | Resident Medical Officer | SMO | Senior Medical Officer |
| TL | Team Leader | Reg | Registrar | E | Emergency Call |

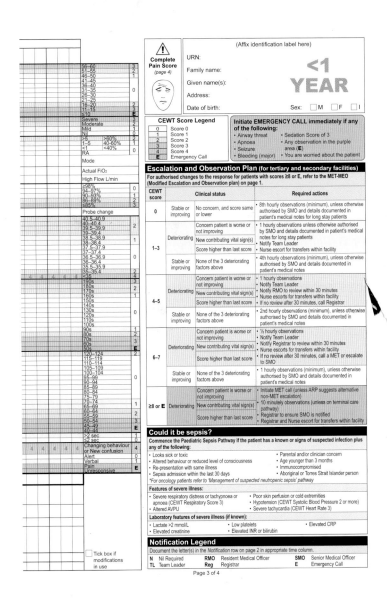

Left column chart (vertical observation chart):

56–60	3
51–55	2
46–50	1
41–45	
36–40	0
31–35	
26–30	
21–25	
16–20	2
11–15	2
≤10	E
Severe	3
Moderate	2
Mild	1
Nil	0
>5 / >60%	2
1–5 / 40–60%	1
<1 / <40%	0
RA	
Mode	
Actual FiO₂	
High Flow L/min	
>98%	0
94–97%	
90–93%	1
86–89%	2
85%	3
Probe change	
40.5–40.9	
40–40.4	2
39.5–39.9	
39–39.4	
38.5–38.9	1
38–38.4	
37.5–37.9	
37–37.4	
36.5–36.9	0
36–36.4	
35.5–35.9	
35–35.4	
<35	2
190s	4
180s	3
170s	2
160s	1
150s	
140s	
130s	0
120s	
110s	
100s	
90s	1
80s	2
70s	3
60s	E
50s	
120–124	2
115–119	
110–114	
105–109	
100–104	0
95–99	
90–94	
85–89	
80–84	
75–79	
70–74	1
65–69	
60–64	2
55–59	
50–54	3
45–49	E
>2 sec	1
≤2 sec	0
Changing behaviour or New confusion	4
Alert	0
Verbal	1
Pain	
Unresponsive	E

☐ Tick box if modifications in use

Pain and Sedation Assessment

- If you are concerned about the patient's pain or sedation but they do not fit the below criteria notify Medical Officer
- For any score in coloured zone follow instructions in action box
- Complete Sedation Score for patients receiving opioids or potentially sedating medication
- Sedation Score is not for use with procedural sedation
- **If an analgesic infusion/bolus is in use, use Paediatric Analgesic Infusion Monitoring Tool**

(Affix identification label here)

URN:

Family name:

Given name(s):

Address:

Date of birth: Sex: ☐ M ☐ F ☐ I

<1 YEAR

Pain Assessment Tools Select (with tick) appropriate pain assessment tool

☐ **FLACC**

Each category is scored 0–2, resulting in a total score of 0–10

Categories	Score 0	Score 1	Score 2
Face	No particular expression or smile	Occasional grimace or frown, withdrawn, disinterested	Frequent to constant frown, clenched jaw, quivering chin
Legs	Normal position, or relaxed	Uneasy, restless, tense	Kicking, or legs drawn up
Activity	Lying quietly, normal position, moves easily	Squirming, shifting back and forth, tense	Arched, rigid, or jerking
Cry	No cry (awake or asleep)	Moans or whimpers, occasional complaint	Crying steadily, screams or sobs, frequent complaints
Consolability	Content, relaxed	Reassured by occasional touching, hugging, or being talked to, distractible	Difficult to console or comfort

	Date															
If Pain and FAS Score conflict follow highest score	Time															

Pain Assessment Chart

• Urgent registrar review. Consider opioids. Obtain a Full CEWT Score. Notify Team Leader. • Contact Acute Pain Service if pain remains severe after permitted interventions	10															
	9															
	8															
• Administer prescribed analgesia • Consider a Full CEWT Score • Registrar review if no improvement • Consider referral to Acute Pain Service if interventions ineffective	7															
	6															
	5															
	4															
• Consider prescribed analgesia • Ward doctor review to prescribe if required	3															
	2															
	1															
• No action	0															

Functional Activity Score (FAS)	Severe	C															
☐ Follow actions for Pain Score 8–10	Mild to Moderate	B															
☐ Follow actions for Pain Score 4–7	Unlimited	A															
Pain relief given		✓															

Sedation Score

• For patients receiving **opioids/potentially sedating medication**	0																
	1																
• Patient **must** be woken to assess Sedation Score • Note: **DO NOT** add the Sedation Score to the CEWT Score. Follow actions below.	2																
	3																

Score	Description	Action
0 or 1	Awake and alert or Easy to rouse, stays awake for ≥10 seconds	• Check Sedation Score before administering opioids/potentially sedating medication • Check Sedation Score 1 hour post administering opioids/potentially sedating medication when it is: » short acting; or » a new medication; or » an increased dose.
2	Easy to rouse but difficulty staying awake, falls asleep <10 seconds	• Ensure patient receives continuous oximetry monitoring and administer oxygen if oxygen saturations <94% • Withhold additional opioids/potentially sedating medication (until medical review) • Notify Team Leader • Notify Medical Officer who must review within 15 mins (remain with the patient until review) • Monitor CEWT and Sedation Score (minimum 15 minutely) until Sedation Score is less than 2 • If concerned, initiate **Emergency Call**
3	Difficult to rouse or unrousable	• Initiate **EMERGENCY CALL** • Ensure patient receives continuous oximetry monitoring and administer oxygen if oxygen saturations <94% • Administer naloxone as per order (for opioids) • Withhold additional opioids/potentially sedating medication • **Monitor CEWT and Sedation Score (minimum 5 minutely) until Sedation Score is less than 3**

References: Merkel et al. (1997). The FLACC: A behavioural scale for scoring postoperative pain in young children. Pediatric Nursing 23(3), 293-297. © 2002. The Regents of the University of Michigan. All rights reserved.

DO NOT WRITE IN THIS BINDING MARGIN

Figure 6.4, *continued*

Queensland Government	(Affix identification label here)
Children's Early Warning Tool (CEWT®)	URN:
	Family name:
1–4 YEARS For tertiary and secondary facilities	Given name(s):
	Address:
Facility:	Date of birth: Sex: ☐ M ☐ F ☐ I

1–4 YEARS

General Instructions

- Full CEWT Score = Respiratory Rate + Respiratory Distress + O_2 + O_2 Saturation + Temperature + Heart Rate + Blood Pressure + Capillary Refill Time + Behaviour and Consciousness.
- A Full CEWT Score and a Pain Score (p4) must be calculated:
  - » on admission
  - » once per 24 hours
  - » if patient is deteriorating or you are concerned.
- A CEWT Score (with BP as clinically indicated) and Pain Score must be calculated at least every 8 hours.
- A Sedation Score must be completed for patients receiving opioids or potentially sedating medication at a clinically appropriate frequency, including prior to administration.
- When graphing observations, place a dot (•) in the appropriate box and join to the preceding dot (e.g. •—•). For blood pressure, use the symbols indicated ($^{\vee}_{\wedge}$).
- Any observation outside the range of the graph, you must write the number.
- Add up all observation scores to calculate the Total CEWT Score and record this in the Total CEWT Score row, even if the score is zero.
- For abnormal observations, you must continue to check until normal.
- Aside from the above, do appropriate observations at an appropriate frequency for the patient's clinical status
- Refer to the table on page 1 for documenting and escalating Changing behaviour.

Date: / /	Time (24hr): :	Random blood glucose level: mmol/L	Is BGL <3 or >8mmol/L? ○ Yes (consult Medical Officer immediately) ☐ No	Blood ketones: mmol/L
Date: / /	Time (24hr): :	Random blood glucose level: mmol/L	Is BGL <3 or >8mmol/L? ○ Yes (consult Medical Officer immediately) ☐ No	Blood ketones: mmol/L

Guide for Recognising Changing Behaviour and New Confusion (page 2)	**Guide for Responding to Changing Behaviour and New Confusion**
• Reported or observed change • Distress • Loss of touch with reality • Loss of function • Elevated risk to self, others, or property	• Changing Behaviour or New Confusion can be a sign of deteriorating psychology or physiology • Escalate as per local protocol (e.g. to speciality Medical or Psychiatry) • If required, activate a Code Black

Interventions

If an intervention is administered, record **here** and note letter in *Interventions* row over page in appropriate time column	A
	B
	C
	D
	E
	F
	G
	H
	I
	J
	K
	L

Height: cm	Weight: kg	Date: / /	Weight: kg	Date: / /	Weight: kg	Date: / /

CEWT® 1–4 YEARS TERTIARY AND SECONDARY

DO NOT WRITE IN THIS BINDING MARGIN

v10.00 - 03/2023
WINC Code: 1NY31745
SW146

CEWT 1–4 Years Old		Date																			
		Time																				
Respiratory Rate (breaths/min) Measure for a full minute	3	51–55																				
	2	46–50																				
	1	41–45																				
		36–40																				
	0	31–35																				
		26–30																				
		21–25																				
	2	16–20																				
	3	11–15																				
		6–10																				
	E	≤5																				
Respiratory Distress	3	Severe																				
	2	Moderate																				
	1	Mild																				
	0	Nil																				
Oxygen* (L/min or % delivered) *If on HF/NIV use % delivered*	2	>5	>60%																			
	1	1–5	40-60%																			
		<1	<40%																			
	0		RA																			
FM Face Mask NP Nasal Prongs HF High Flow NRM Non Re-breather Mask NIV Non invasive RA Room Air		Mode																				
Actual FiO₂ on Device Screen																						
High Flow L/min on Device Screen																						
O₂ Saturation (%)	0	>98%																				
		94–97%																				
	1	90–93%																				
	2	86–89%																				
	3	≤85%																				
Probe change																						
Temperature (°C)		40.5–40.9																				
	2	40–40.4																				
		39.5–39.9																				
		39–39.4																				
	1	38.5–38.9																				
		38–38.4																				
		37.5–37.9																				
	0	37–37.4																				
		36.5–36.9																				
		36–36.4																				
		35.5–35.9																				
	2	35–35.4																				
	4	<35																				
Heart Rate (beats/min)	3	170s																				
	2	160s																				
		150s																				
	1	140s																				
		130s																				
	0	120s																				
		110s																				
		100s																				
		90s																				
	1	80s																				
	2	70s																				
	3	60s																				
	E	50s																				
Blood Pressure (mmHg) **Score systolic BP**	2	125–129																				
		120–124																				
		115–119																				
		110–114																				
		105–109																				
	0	100–104																				
		95–99																				
		90–94																				
		85–89																				
		80–84																				
	1	75–79																				
		70–74																				
	2	65–69																				
	3	60–64																				
		55–59																				
	E	50–54																				
		45–49																				
Capillary Refill Time	1	>2 sec																				
	0	≤2 sec																				
Behaviour and Consciousness If necessary, wake patient before scoring	4	Changing behaviour or New confusion																				
	0	Alert																				
	1	Voice																				
		Pain																				
	E	Unresponsive																				
Total CEWT Score																						
SMO authorised change to observation frequencies in place *Refer to patient's medical notes for details*	SMO																					
MET-MEO (Modified Escalation and Observation) Plan in place	MEO																					
Notification (most senior position, see legend on pg3)																						
Is Plan in place for managing Changing behaviour or New Confusion? *If Plan in place to manage Changing Behaviour or New Confusion, score AVPU as usual*	Y OR N																					
Interventions	(e.g. A)																					
Initials																						

Page 2 of 4

Figure 6.4, *continued*

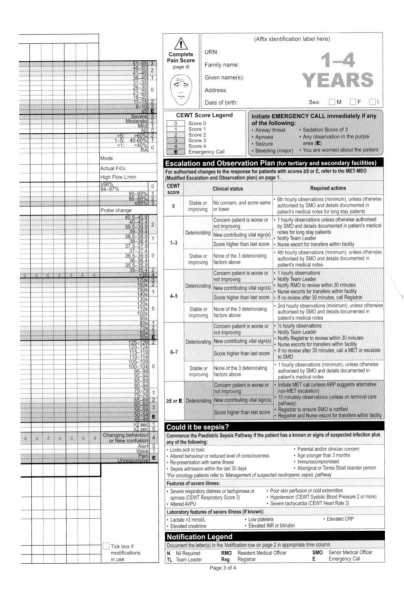

Complete Pain Score (page 4)

(Affix identification label here)

URN:

Family name:

Given name(s):

Address:

Date of birth:

Sex: ☐ M ☐ F ☐ I

1–4 YEARS

CEWT Score Legend

0	Score 0
1	Score 1
2	Score 2
3	Score 3
4	Score 4
E	Emergency Call

Initiate EMERGENCY CALL immediately if any of the following:
- Airway threat
- Apnoea
- Seizure
- Bleeding (major)
- Sedation Score of 3
- Any observation in the purple area (**E**)
- You are worried about the patient

Escalation and Observation Plan (for tertiary and secondary facilities)

For authorised changes to the response for patients with scores ≥8 or E, refer to the MET-MEO (Modified Escalation and Observation plan) on page 1.

CEWT score		Clinical status	Required actions
0	Stable or improving	No concern, and score same or lower	• 8th hourly observations (minimum), unless otherwise authorised by SMO and details documented in patient's medical notes for long stay patients
1–3	Deteriorating	Concern patient is worse or not improving	• 1 hourly observations unless otherwise authorised by SMO and details documented in patient's medical notes for long stay patients
		New contributing vital sign(s)	• Notify Team Leader
		Score higher than last score	• Nurse escort for transfers within facility
	Stable or improving	None of the 3 deteriorating factors above	• 4th hourly observations (minimum), unless otherwise authorised by SMO and details documented in patient's medical notes
4–5	Deteriorating	Concern patient is worse or not improving	• 1 hourly observations
		New contributing vital sign(s)	• Notify Team Leader
			• Notify RMO to review within 30 minutes
		Score higher than last score	• Nurse escorts for transfers within facility
			• If no review after 30 minutes, call Registrar
	Stable or improving	None of the 3 deteriorating factors above	• 2nd hourly observations (minimum), unless otherwise authorised by SMO and details documented in patient's medical notes
6–7	Deteriorating	Concern patient is worse or not improving	• ½ hourly observations
		New contributing vital sign(s)	• Notify Team Leader
			• Notify Registrar to review within 30 minutes
		Score higher than last score	• Nurse escorts for transfers within facility
			• If no review after 30 minutes, call a MET or escalate to SMO
	Stable or improving	None of the 3 deteriorating factors above	• 1 hourly observations (minimum), unless otherwise authorised by SMO and details documented in patient's medical notes
≥8 or E	Deteriorating	Concern patient is worse or not improving	• Initiate MET call (unless ARP suggests alternative non-MET escalation)
		New contributing vital sign(s)	• 10 minutely observations (unless on terminal care pathway)
		Score higher than last score	• Registrar to ensure SMO is notified
			• Registrar and Nurse escort for transfers within facility

Could it be sepsis?

Commence the Paediatric Sepsis Pathway if the patient has a known or signs of suspected infection plus any of the following:
- Looks sick or toxic
- Altered behaviour or reduced level of consciousness
- Re-presentation with same illness
- Sepsis admission within the last 30 days
- Parental and/or clinician concern
- Age younger than 3 months
- Immunocompromised
- Aboriginal or Torres Strait Islander person

*For oncology patients refer to 'Management of suspected neutropenic sepsis' pathway

Features of severe illness:
- Severe respiratory distress or tachypnoea or apnoea (CEWT Respiratory Score 3)
- Altered AVPU
- Poor skin perfusion or cold extremities
- Hypotension (CEWT Systolic Blood Pressure 2 or more)
- Severe tachycardia (CEWT Heart Rate 3)

Laboratory features of severe illness (if known):
- Lactate >2 mmol/L
- Elevated creatinine
- Low platelets
- Elevated INR or bilirubin
- Elevated CRP

Notification Legend

Document the letter(s) in the *Notification* row on page 2 in appropriate time column.

N	Nil Required	RMO	Resident Medical Officer	SMO	Senior Medical Officer
TL	Team Leader	Reg	Registrar	E	Emergency Call

Tick box if modifications in use

Pain and Sedation Assessment

- If you are concerned about the patient's pain or sedation but they do not fit the below criteria notify Medical Officer
- For any score in coloured zone follow instructions in action box
- Complete Sedation Score for patients receiving opioids or potentially sedating medication
- Sedation Score is not for use with procedural sedation
- **If an analgesic infusion/bolus is in use, use Paediatric Analgesic Infusion Monitoring Tool**

(Affix identification label here)

URN:

Family name:

Given name(s):

Address:

Date of birth: Sex: ☐ M ☐ F ☐ I

1–4 YEARS

Pain Assessment Tools Select (with tick) appropriate pain assessment tool

☐ The Faces Pain Scale - Revised (FPS-R) 4+ years Use laminated card	"These faces show how much something can hurt. This face [point to left-most face] shows no pain. The faces show more and more pain [point to each from left to right] up to this one [point to right-most face] - it shows very much pain. Point to the face that shows how much you hurt [right now]."

0   2   4   6   8   10

☐ FLACC 15 days to 3 years *(or as required)* Each category is scored 0 to 2 resulting in a total score of 0 to 10	Categories	Score 0	Score 1	Score 2
	Face	No particular expression or smile	Occasional grimace or frown, withdrawn, disinterested	Frequent to constant frown, clenched jaw, quivering chin
	Legs	Normal position, or relaxed	Uneasy, restless, tense	Kicking, or legs drawn up
	Activity	Lying quietly, normal position, moves easily	Squirming, shifting back and forth, tense	Arched, rigid, or jerking
	Cry	No cry (awake or asleep)	Moans or whimpers, occasional complaint	Crying steadily, screams or sobs, frequent complaints
	Consolability	Content, relaxed	Reassured by occasional touching, hugging, or being talked to, distractible	Difficult to console or comfort

If Pain and FAS Score conflict follow highest score

Date													
Time													

Pain Assessment Chart

• Urgent registrar review. Consider opioids. Obtain a Full CEWT Score. Notify Team Leader. • Contact Acute Pain Service if pain remains severe after permitted interventions	10													
	9													
	8													
• Administer prescribed analgesia • Consider a Full CEWT Score • Registrar review if no improvement • Consider referral to Acute Pain Service if interventions ineffective	7													
	6													
	5													
	4													
• Consider prescribed analgesia • Ward doctor review to prescribe if required	3													
	2													
	1													
• No action	0													

Functional Activity Score (FAS)

☐ Follow actions for Pain Score 8–10	Severe	C												
☐ Follow actions for Pain Score 4–7	Mild to Moderate	B												
	Unlimited	A												
Pain relief given		✓												

Sedation Score

• For patients receiving **opioids/potentially sedating medication**	0													
• Patient **must** be woken to assess Sedation Score	1													
• Note: **DO NOT** add the Sedation Score to the CEWT Score. Follow actions below.	2													
	3													

Score	Description	Action
0 *or* 1	Awake and alert *or* Easy to rouse, stays awake for ≥10 seconds	• Check Sedation Score before administering opioids/potentially sedating medication • Check Sedation Score 1 hour post administering opioids/potentially sedating medication when it is: » short acting; *or* » a new medication; *or* » an increased dose.
2	Easy to rouse but difficulty staying awake, falls asleep <10 seconds	• Ensure patient receives continuous oximetry monitoring and administer oxygen if oxygen saturations <94% • Withhold additional opioids/potentially sedating medication (until medical review) • Notify Team Leader • Notify Medical Officer who must review within 15 mins (remain with the patient until review) • Monitor CEWT and Sedation Score (minimum 15 minutely) until Sedation Score is less than 2 • If concerned, initiate **Emergency Call**
3	Difficult to rouse or unrousable	• Initiate **EMERGENCY CALL** • Ensure patient receives continuous oximetry monitoring and administer oxygen if oxygen saturations <94% • Administer naloxone as per order *(for opioids)* • Withhold additional opioids/potentially sedating medication • **Monitor CEWT and Sedation Score (minimum 5 minutely) until Sedation Score is less than 3**

References: FPS-R: Hicks CL et al., PAIN 2001;93:173. ©2001 International Association for the Study of Pain, reproduced with permission. www.iasp-pain.org/FPSR. Merkel et al. (1997). The FLACC: A behavioural scale for scoring postoperative pain in young children. Pediatric Nursing 23(3), 293-297. © 2002, The Regents of the University of Michigan. All rights reserved.

DO NOT WRITE IN THIS BINDING MARGIN

Figure 6.4, *continued*

Queensland Government **Children's Early Warning Tool (CEWT®)** **5–11 YEARS** For tertiary and secondary facilities	(Affix identification label here)
	URN:
	Family name: **5–11 YEARS**
	Given name(s):
	Address:
Facility:	Date of birth: Sex: ☐ M ☐ F ☐ I

General Instructions

- Full CEWT Score = Respiratory Rate + Respiratory Distress + O₂ + O₂ Saturation + Temperature + Heart Rate + Blood Pressure + Capillary Refill Time + Behaviour and Consciousness.
- A Full CEWT Score and a Pain Score (p4) must be calculated:
  - » on admission
  - » once per 24 hours
  - » if patient is deteriorating or you are concerned.
- A CEWT Score (with BP as clinically indicated) and Pain Score must be calculated at least every 8 hours.
- A Sedation Score must be completed for patients receiving opioids or potentially sedating medication at a clinically appropriate frequency, including prior to administration.
- When graphing observations, place a dot (•) in the appropriate box and join to the preceding dot (e.g. ⌒). For blood pressure, use the symbols indicated (⊻).
- Any observation outside the range of the graph, you must write the number.
- Add up all observation scores to calculate the Total CEWT Score and record this in the Total CEWT Score row, even if the score is zero.
- For abnormal observations, you must continue to check until normal.
- Aside from the above, do appropriate observations at an appropriate frequency for the patient's clinical status
- Refer to the table on page 1 for documenting and escalating Changing behaviour.

Date: / /	Time (24hr): :	Random blood glucose level: mmol/L	Is BGL <3 or >8mmol/L? ☐ Yes (consult Medical Officer immediately) ☐ No	Blood ketones: mmol/L
Date: / /	Time (24hr): :	Random blood glucose level: mmol/L	Is BGL <3 or >8mmol/L? ☐ Yes (consult Medical Officer immediately) ☐ No	Blood ketones: mmol/L

Guide for Recognising Changing Behaviour and New Confusion (page 2)	**Guide for Responding to Changing Behaviour and New Confusion**
• Reported or observed change • Distress • Loss of touch with reality • Loss of function • Elevated risk to self, others, or property	• Changing Behaviour or New Confusion can be a sign of deteriorating psychology or physiology • Escalate as per local protocol (e.g. to speciality Medical or Psychiatry) • If required, activate a Code Black

Interventions

If an intervention is administered, record **here** and note letter in *Interventions* row over page in appropriate time column	A
	B
	C
	D
	E
	F
	G
	H
	I
	J
	K
	L

Height: cm	Weight: kg Date: / /	Weight: kg Date: / /	Weight: kg Date: / /

CEWT® 5–11 YEARS   TERTIARY AND SECONDARY

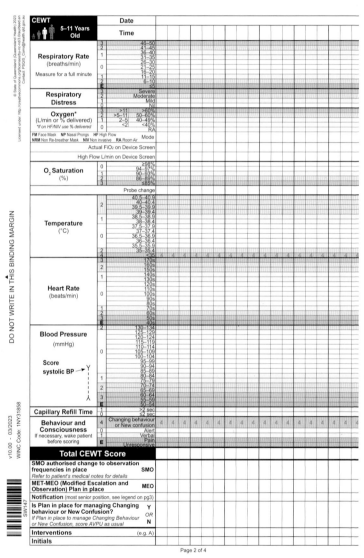

Figure 6.4, *continued*

(Affix identification label here)

URN:

Family name:

Given name(s):

Address:

Date of birth: Sex: ☐ M ☐ F ☐ I

5–11 YEARS

Complete Pain Score (page 4)		

CEWT Score Legend

0	Score 0
1	Score 1
2	Score 2
3	Score 3
4	Score 4
E	Emergency Call

Initiate EMERGENCY CALL immediately if any of the following:

- Airway threat
- Apnoea
- Seizure
- Bleeding (major)
- Sedation Score of 3
- Any observation in the purple area (**E**)
- You are worried about the patient

Escalation and Observation Plan (for tertiary and secondary facilities)

For authorised changes to the response for patients with scores ≥8 or E, refer to the MET-MEO (Modified Escalation and Observation plan) on page 1.

CEWT score	Clinical status		Required actions
0	Stable or improving	No concern, and score same or lower	• 8th hourly observations (minimum), unless otherwise authorised by SMO and details documented in patient's medical notes for long stay patients
1–3	Deteriorating	Concern patient is worse or not improving	• 1 hourly observations unless otherwise authorised by SMO and details documented in patient's medical notes for long stay patients • Notify Team Leader • Nurse escort for transfers within facility
		New contributing vital sign(s)	
		Score higher than last score	
	Stable or improving	None of the 3 deteriorating factors above	• 4th hourly observations, unless otherwise authorised by SMO and details documented in patient's medical notes
4–5	Deteriorating	Concern patient is worse or not improving	• 1 hourly observations • Notify Team Leader • Notify RMO to review within 30 minutes • Nurse escorts for transfers within facility • If no review after 30 minutes, call Registrar
		New contributing vital sign(s)	
		Score higher than last score	
	Stable or improving	None of the 3 deteriorating factors above	• 2nd hourly observations (minimum), unless otherwise authorised by SMO and details documented in patient's medical notes
6–7	Deteriorating	Concern patient is worse or not improving	• ½ hourly observations • Notify Team Leader • Notify Registrar to review within 30 minutes • Nurse escorts for transfers within facility • If no review after 30 minutes, call a MET or escalate to SMO
		New contributing vital sign(s)	
		Score higher than last score	
	Stable or improving	None of the 3 deteriorating factors above	• 1 hourly observations (minimum), unless otherwise authorised by SMO and details documented in patient's medical notes
≥8 or **E**	Deteriorating	Concern patient is worse or not improving	• Initiate MET call (unless ARP suggests alternative non-MET escalation) • 10 minutely observations (unless on terminal care pathway) • Registrar to ensure SMO is notified • Registrar and Nurse escort for transfers within facility
		New contributing vital sign(s)	
		Score higher than last score	

Could it be sepsis?

Commence the Paediatric Sepsis Pathway if the patient has a known or signs of suspected infection plus any of the following:

- Looks sick or toxic
- Altered behaviour or reduced level of consciousness
- Re-presentation with same illness
- Sepsis admission within the last 30 days
- Parental and/or clinician concern
- Age younger than 3 months
- Immunocompromised
- Aboriginal or Torres Strait Islander person

For oncology patients refer to 'Management of suspected neutropenic sepsis' pathway

Features of severe illness:

- Severe respiratory distress or tachypnoea or apnoea (CEWT Respiratory Score 3)
- Altered AVPU
- Poor skin perfusion or cold extremities
- Hypotension (CEWT Systolic Blood Pressure 2 or more)
- Severe tachycardia (CEWT Heart Rate 3)

Laboratory features of severe illness (if known):

- Lactate >2 mmol/L
- Elevated creatinine
- Low platelets
- Elevated INR or bilirubin
- Elevated CRP

Notification Legend

Document the letter(s) in the *Notification* row on page 2 in appropriate time column.

N	Nil Required	RMO	Resident Medical Officer	SMO	Senior Medical Officer
TL	Team Leader	Reg	Registrar	E	Emergency Call

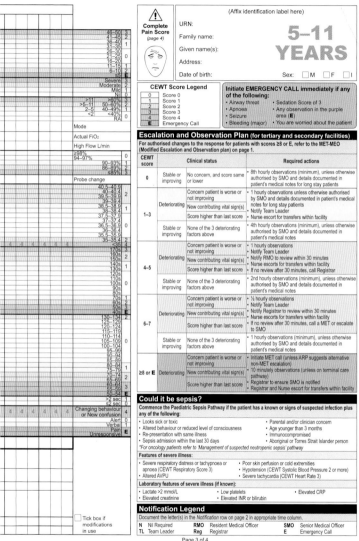

Left-hand observation chart columns:

46–50	3
41–45	2
36–40	1
31–35	0
26–30	
21–25	0
16–20	
11–15	1
6–10	2
<5	E

Severe	3
Moderate	2
Mild	1
Nil	0

>11	>60%	3
>5–11	50–60%	2
2–5	40–49%	1
<2	<40%	0
	RA	

Mode

Actual FiO₂

High Flow L/min

>98%	0
94–97%	
90–93%	1
86–89%	2
≤85%	3

Probe change

40.5–40.9	
40.0–40.4	2
39.5–39.9	
39.0–39.4	
38.5–38.9	1
38.0–38.4	
37.5–37.9	
37.0–37.4	
36.5–36.9	0
36.0–36.4	
35.5–35.9	
35.0–35.4	2
<35	4

170s	3
160s	2
150s	
140s	1
130s	
120s	
110s	
100s	0
90s	
80s	
70s	1
60s	2
50s	3
40s	E

130–134	2
125–129	
120–124	
115–119	
110–114	
105–109	0
100–104	
95–99	
90–94	
85–89	
80–84	1
75–79	
70–74	2
65–69	
60–64	3
55–59	
50–54	E

| >2 sec | 1 |
| <2 sec | 0 |

Changing behaviour or New confusion	4
Alert	0
Verbal	1
Pain	
Unresponsive	E

☐ Tick box if modifications in use

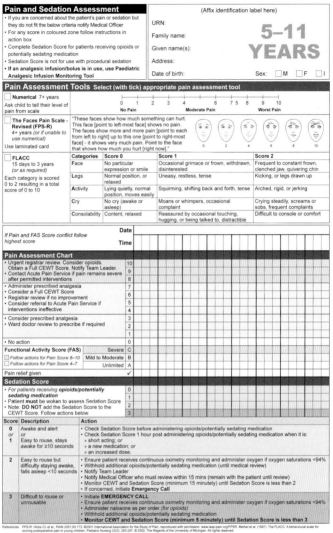

Pain and Sedation Assessment

- If you are concerned about the patient's pain or sedation but they do not fit the below criteria notify Medical Officer
- For any score in coloured zone follow instructions in action box
- Complete Sedation Score for patients receiving opioids or potentially sedating medication
- Sedation Score is not for use with procedural sedation
- **If an analgesic infusion/bolus is in use, use Paediatric Analgesic Infusion Monitoring Tool**

(Affix identification label here)

URN:
Family name:
Given name(s):
Address:
Date of birth: Sex: ☐ M ☐ F ☐ I

5–11 YEARS

Pain Assessment Tools Select (with tick) appropriate pain assessment tool

☐ **Numerical** 7+ years
Ask child to tell their level of pain from scale

0	1	2	3	4		6	7	8	9	10
No Pain				Moderate Pain						Worst Pain

☐ **The Faces Pain Scale - Revised (FPS-R)**
4+ years (or if unable to use numerical)
Use laminated card

"These faces show how much something can hurt. This face [point to left-most face] shows no pain. The faces show more and more pain [point to each from left to right] up to this one [point to right-most face] - it shows very much pain. Point to the face that shows how much you hurt [right now]."

0   2   4   6   8   10

☐ **FLACC**
15 days to 3 years (or as required)
Each category is scored 0 to 2 resulting in a total score of 0 to 10

Categories	Score 0	Score 1	Score 2
Face	No particular expression or smile	Occasional grimace or frown, withdrawn, disinterested	Frequent to constant frown, clenched jaw, quivering chin
Legs	Normal position, or relaxed	Uneasy, restless, tense	Kicking, or legs drawn up
Activity	Lying quietly, normal position, moves easily	Squirming, shifting back and forth, tense	Arched, rigid, or jerking
Cry	No cry (awake or asleep)	Moans or whimpers, occasional complaint	Crying steadily, screams or sobs, frequent complaints
Consolability	Content, relaxed	Reassured by occasional touching, hugging, or being talked to, distractible	Difficult to console or comfort

If Pain and FAS Score conflict follow highest score

	Date													
	Time													

Pain Assessment Chart

• Urgent registrar review. Consider opioids. Obtain a Full CEWT Score. Notify Team Leader. • Contact Acute Pain Service if pain remains severe after permitted interventions	10													
	9													
	8													
• Administer prescribed analgesia • Consider a Full CEWT Score • Registrar review if no improvement • Consider referral to Acute Pain Service if interventions ineffective	7													
	6													
	5													
	4													
• Consider prescribed analgesia • Ward doctor review to prescribe if required	3													
	2													
	1													
• No action	0													

Functional Activity Score (FAS)	Severe	C													
☐ *Follow actions for Pain Score 8–10*	Mild to Moderate	B													
☐ *Follow actions for Pain Score 4–7*	Unlimited	A													
Pain relief given		✓													

Sedation Score

• For patients receiving **opioids/potentially sedating medication** • Patient **must** be woken to assess Sedation Score • Note: **DO NOT** add the Sedation Score to the CEWT Score. Follow actions below.	0													
	1													
	2													
	3													

Score	Description	Action
0 or 1	Awake and alert / Easy to rouse, stays awake for ≥10 seconds	• Check Sedation Score before administering opioids/potentially sedating medication • Check Sedation Score 1 hour post administering opioids/potentially sedating medication when it is: » short acting; or » a new medication; or » an increased dose.
2	Easy to rouse but difficulty staying awake, falls asleep <10 seconds	• Ensure patient receives continuous oximetry monitoring and administer oxygen if oxygen saturations <94% • Withhold additional opioids/potentially sedating medication (until medical review) • Notify Team Leader • Notify Medical Officer who must review within 15 mins (remain with the patient until review) • Monitor CEWT and Sedation Score (minimum 15 minutely) until Sedation Score is less than 2 • If concerned, initiate **Emergency Call**
3	Difficult to rouse or unrousable	• Initiate **EMERGENCY CALL** • Ensure patient receives continuous oximetry monitoring and administer oxygen if oxygen saturations <94% • Administer naloxone as per order (for opioids) • Withhold additional opioids/potentially sedating medication • **Monitor CEWT and Sedation Score (minimum 5 minutely) until Sedation Score is less than 3**

Page 4 of 4

DO NOT WRITE IN THIS BINDING MARGIN

Figure 6.4, *continued*

Queensland Government

Children's Early Warning Tool (CEWT®)

12–17 YEARS
For tertiary and secondary facilities

Facility:

(Affix identification label here)

URN:

Family name:

Given name(s):

Address:

Date of birth: Sex: ☐ M ☐ F ☐ I

12–17 YEARS

General Instructions

- Full CEWT Score = Respiratory Rate + Respiratory Distress + O_2 + O_2 Saturation + Temperature + Heart Rate +
  Blood Pressure + Capillary Refill Time + Behaviour and Consciousness.
- A Full CEWT Score and a Pain Score (p4) must be calculated:
  - » on admission
  - » once per 24 hours
  - » if patient is deteriorating or you are concerned.
- A CEWT Score (with BP as clinically indicated) and Pain Score must be calculated at least every 8 hours.
- A Sedation Score must be completed for patients receiving opioids or potentially sedating medication at a clinically appropriate frequency, including prior to administration.
- When graphing observations, place a dot (•) in the appropriate box and join to the preceding dot (e.g. ⌐•). For blood pressure, use the symbols indicated (Y ∧).
- Any observation outside the range of the graph, you must write the number.
- Add up all observation scores to calculate the Total CEWT Score and record this in the Total CEWT Score row, even if score is zero.
- For abnormal observations, you must continue to check until normal.
- Aside from the above, do appropriate observations at an appropriate frequency for the patient's clinical status
- Refer to the table on page 1 for documenting and escalating Changing behaviour.

Date:	Time (24hr):	Random blood glucose level:	Is BGL <3 or >8mmol/L?	Blood ketones:
/ /	:	mmol/L	◯ **Yes** (consult Medical Officer immediately) ☐ No	mmol/L
Date:	Time (24hr):	Random blood glucose level:	Is BGL <3 or >8mmol/L?	Blood ketones:
/ /	:	mmol/L	◯ **Yes** (consult Medical Officer immediately) ☐ No	mmol/L

Guide for Recognising Changing Behaviour and New Confusion (page 2)

- Reported or observed change
- Distress
- Loss of touch with reality
- Loss of function
- Elevated risk to self, others, or property

Guide for Responding to Changing Behaviour and New Confusion

- Changing Behaviour or New Confusion can be a sign of deteriorating psychology or physiology
- Escalate as per local protocol (e.g. to speciality Medical or Psychiatry)
- If required, activate a Code Black

Interventions

If an intervention is administered, record **here** and note letter in *Interventions* row over page in appropriate time column

A	
B	
C	
D	
E	
F	
G	
H	
I	
J	
K	
L	

Height:	Weight:	Date:	Weight:	Date:	Weight:	Date:
cm	kg	/ /	kg	/ /	kg	/ /

CEWT® 12–17 YEARS

TERTIARY AND SECONDARY

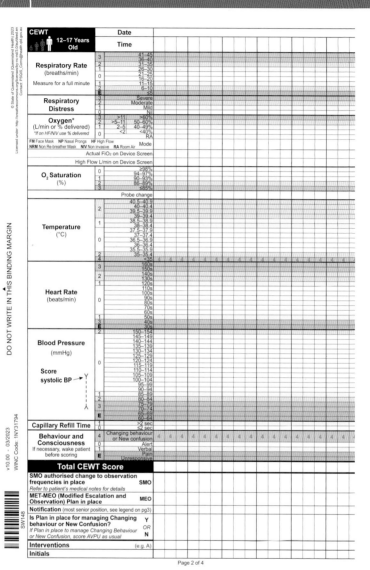

DO NOT WRITE IN THIS BINDING MARGIN

v10.00 – 03/2023
WINC Code: 1NY31794
SW148

CEWT 12–17 Years Old		Date																	
		Time																	
Respiratory Rate (breaths/min) Measure for a full minute	3	41–45																	
	2	36–40																	
	1	31–35																	
		26–30																	
	0	21–25																	
		16–20																	
	1	11–15																	
	2	6–10																	
	E	≤5																	
Respiratory Distress	3	Severe																	
	2	Moderate																	
	1	Mild																	
	0	Nil																	
Oxygen* (L/min or % delivered) *If on HF/NIV use % delivered*	3	>11	>60%																
	2	>5–11	50–60%																
	1	2–5	40–49%																
		<2	<40%																
	0		RA																
FM Face Mask NP Nasal Prongs HF High Flow NRM Non Re-breather Mask NIV Non invasive RA Room Air		Mode																	
		Actual FiO₂ on Device Screen																	
		High Flow L/min on Device Screen																	
O₂ Saturation (%)	0	≥98%																	
		94–97%																	
	1	90–93%																	
	2	86–89%																	
	3	≤85%																	
		Probe change																	
Temperature (°C)		40.5–40.9																	
	2	40–40.4																	
		39.5–39.9																	
		39–39.4																	
	1	38.5–38.9																	
		38–38.4																	
		37.5–37.9																	
	0	37–37.4																	
		36.5–36.9																	
		36–36.4																	
		35.5–35.9																	
	2	35–35.4																	
	4	<35																	
Heart Rate (beats/min)	3	160s																	
		150s																	
	2	140s																	
		130s																	
	1	120s																	
		110s																	
		100s																	
	0	90s																	
		80s																	
		70s																	
		60s																	
	1	50s																	
	3	40s																	
	E	30s																	
Blood Pressure (mmHg) Score systolic BP	2	150–154																	
		145–149																	
		140–144																	
		135–139																	
		130–134																	
		125–129																	
	0	120–124																	
		115–119																	
		110–114																	
		105–109																	
		100–104																	
		95–99																	
		90–94																	
	1	85–89																	
	2	80–84																	
	3	75–79																	
		70–74																	
	E	65–69																	
		60–64																	
Capillary Refill Time	0	>2 sec																	
		≤2 sec																	
Behaviour and Consciousness If necessary, wake patient before scoring	4	Changing behaviour or New confusion																	
	0	Alert																	
	1	Verbal																	
		Pain																	
	E	Unresponsive																	
Total CEWT Score																			
SMO authorised change to observation frequencies in place *Refer to patient's medical notes for details*	SMO																		
MET-MEO (Modified Escalation and Observation) Plan in place	MEO																		
Notification (most senior position, see legend on pg3)																			
Is Plan in place for managing Changing behaviour or New Confusion? *If Plan in place to manage Changing Behaviour or New Confusion, score AVPU as usual*	Y OR N																		
Interventions (e.g. A)																			
Initials																			

Page 2 of 4

Figure 6.4, *continued*

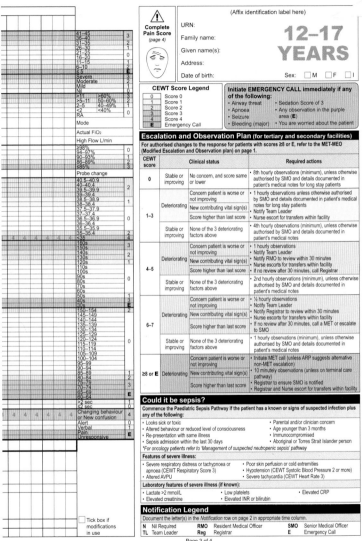

Complete Pain Score *(page 4)*

(Affix identification label here)

URN:
Family name:
Given name(s):
Address:
Date of birth: Sex: ☐ M ☐ F ☐ I

12–17 YEARS

	Scale	
	41–45	3
	36–40	2
	31–35	2
	26–30	1
	21–25	0
	16–20	1
	11–15	1
	6–10	2
	≤ 5	E
	Severe	3
	Moderate	2
	Mild	1
	Nil	0

	>11	>60%	3
	>5–11	50–60%	2
	2–5	40–49%	1
	<2	<40%	0
	RA		

Mode

Actual FiO₂

High Flow L/min

≥98%	0
94–97%	0
90–93%	1
86–89%	2
≤85%	3

Probe change

40.5–40.9	
40–40.4	2
39.5–39.9	
39–39.4	
38.5–38.9	1
38–38.4	
37.5–37.9	
37–37.4	
36.5–36.9	0
36–36.4	
35.5–35.9	
35–35.4	2
<35	3

160s	3
150s	2
140s	
130s	1
120s	
110s	
100s	0
90s	
80s	
70s	
60s	
50s	
40s	1
30s	E
	2

150–154	
145–149	
140–144	
135–139	
130–134	
125–129	
120–124	0
115–119	
110–114	
105–109	
100–104	
95–99	
90–94	
85–89	1
80–84	2
75–79	3
70–74	
65–69	E
60–64	

>2 sec	1
≤2 sec	0
Changing behaviour or New confusion	4
Alert	0
Verbal	1
Pain	
Unresponsive	E

☐ Tick box if modifications in use

CEWT Score Legend

0	Score 0
1	Score 1
2	Score 2
3	Score 3
4	Score 4
E	Emergency Call

Initiate EMERGENCY CALL immediately if any of the following:
- Airway threat
- Apnoea
- Seizure
- Bleeding (major)
- Sedation Score of 3
- Any observation in the purple area (**E**)
- You are worried about the patient

Escalation and Observation Plan (for tertiary and secondary facilities)

For authorised changes to the response for patients with scores ≥8 or E, refer to the MET-MEO (Modified Escalation and Observation plan) on page 1.

CEWT score	Clinical status		Required actions
0	Stable or improving	No concern, and score same or lower	• 8th hourly observations (minimum), unless otherwise authorised by SMO and details documented in patient's medical notes for long stay patients
1–3	Deteriorating	Concern patient is worse or not improving	• 1 hourly observations unless otherwise authorised by SMO and details documented in patient's medical notes for long stay patients
		New contributing vital sign(s)	• Notify Team Leader
		Score higher than last score	• Nurse escort for transfers within facility
	Stable or improving	None of the 3 deteriorating factors above	• 4th hourly observations (minimum), unless otherwise authorised by SMO and details documented in patient's medical notes
4–5	Deteriorating	Concern patient is worse or not improving	• 1 hourly observations
		New contributing vital sign(s)	• Notify Team Leader
			• Notify RMO to review within 30 minutes
		Score higher than last score	• Nurse escorts for transfers within facility
			• If no review after 30 minutes, call Registrar
	Stable or improving	None of the 3 deteriorating factors above	• 2nd hourly observations (minimum), unless otherwise authorised by SMO and details documented in patient's medical notes
6–7	Deteriorating	Concern patient is worse or not improving	• ½ hourly observations
		New contributing vital sign(s)	• Notify Team Leader
			• Notify Registrar to review within 30 minutes
		Score higher than last score	• Nurse escorts for transfers within facility
			• If no review after 30 minutes, call a MET or escalate to SMO
	Stable or improving	None of the 3 deteriorating factors above	• 1 hourly observations (minimum), unless otherwise authorised by SMO and details documented in patient's medical notes
≥8 or E	Deteriorating	Concern patient is worse or not improving	• Initiate MET call (unless ARP suggests alternative non-MET escalation)
		New contributing vital sign(s)	• 10 minutely observations (unless on terminal care pathway)
		Score higher than last score	• Registrar to ensure SMO is notified
			• Registrar and Nurse escort for transfers within facility

Could it be sepsis?

Commence the Paediatric Sepsis Pathway if the patient has a known or signs of suspected infection plus any of the following:
- Looks sick or toxic
- Altered behaviour or reduced level of consciousness
- Re-presentation with same illness
- Sepsis admission within the last 30 days
- Parental and/or clinician concern
- Age younger than 3 months
- Immunocompromised
- Aboriginal or Torres Strait Islander person

*For oncology patients refer to 'Management of suspected neutropenic sepsis' pathway

Features of severe illness:
- Severe respiratory distress or tachypnoea or apnoea (CEWT Respiratory Score 3)
- Altered AVPU
- Poor skin perfusion or cold extremities
- Hypotension (CEWT Systolic Blood Pressure 2 or more)
- Severe tachycardia (CEWT Heart Rate 3)

Laboratory features of severe illness (if known):
- Lactate >2 mmol/L
- Elevated creatinine
- Low platelets
- Elevated INR or bilirubin
- Elevated CRP

Notification Legend

Document the letter(s) in the *Notification* row on page 2 in appropriate time column.

N	Nil Required	RMO	Resident Medical Officer	SMO	Senior Medical Officer
TL	Team Leader	Reg	Registrar	E	Emergency Call

Pain and Sedation Assessment

- If you are concerned about the patient's pain or sedation but they do not fit the below criteria notify Medical Officer
- For any score in coloured zone follow instructions in action box
- Complete Sedation Score for patients receiving opioids or potentially sedating medication
- Sedation Score is not for use with procedural sedation
- **If an analgesic infusion/bolus is in use, use Paediatric Analgesic Infusion Monitoring Tool**

(Affix identification label here)

URN:

Family name:

Given name(s):

Address:

Date of birth: Sex: ☐ M ☐ F ☐ I

12–17 YEARS

Pain Assessment Tools Select (with tick) appropriate pain assessment tool

☐ **Numerical** 7+ years
Ask child to tell their level of pain from scale

| 0 | 1 | 2 | 3 | 4 | 6 | 7 5 | 8 | 9 | 10 |
No Pain   Moderate Pain   Worst Pain

☐ **The Faces Pain Scale - Revised (FPS-R)**
4+ years *(or if unable to use numerical)*
Use laminated card

"These faces show how much something can hurt. This face [point to left-most face] shows no pain. The faces show more and more pain [point to each from left to right] up to this one [point to right-most face] - it shows very much pain. Point to the face that shows how much you hurt [right now]."

| 0 | 2 | 4 | 6 | 8 | 10 |

☐ **FLACC**
15 days to 3 years *(or as required)*
Each category is scored 0 to 2 resulting in a total score of 0 to 10

Categories	Score 0	Score 1	Score 2
Face	No particular expression or smile	Occasional grimace or frown, withdrawn, disinterested	Frequent to constant frown, clenched jaw, quivering chin
Legs	Normal position, or relaxed	Uneasy, restless, tense	Kicking, or legs drawn up
Activity	Lying quietly, normal position, moves easily	Squirming, shifting back and forth, tense	Arched, rigid, or jerking
Cry	No cry (awake or asleep)	Moans or whimpers, occasional complaint	Crying steadily, screams or sobs, frequent complaints
Consolability	Content, relaxed	Reassured by occasional touching, hugging, or being talked to, distractible	Difficult to console or comfort

If Pain and FAS Score conflict follow highest score

	Date													
	Time													

Pain Assessment Chart

- Urgent registrar review. Consider opioids. Obtain a Full CEWT Score. Notify Team Leader.
- Contact Acute Pain Service if pain remains severe after permitted interventions

10														
9														
8														

- Administer prescribed analgesia
- Consider a Full CEWT Score
- Registrar review if no improvement
- Consider referral to Acute Pain Service if interventions ineffective

7														
6														
5														
4														

- Consider prescribed analgesia
- Ward doctor review to prescribe if required

3														
2														
1														

- No action

| 0 | | | | | | | | | | | | | | |

Functional Activity Score (FAS)	Severe	C													
☐ Follow actions for Pain Score 8–10	Mild to Moderate	B													
☐ Follow actions for Pain Score 4–7	Unlimited	A													
Pain relief given		✓													

Sedation Score

- For patients receiving **opioids/potentially sedating medication**
- Patient **must** be woken to assess Sedation Score
- Note: **DO NOT** add the Sedation Score to the CEWT Score. Follow actions below.

0															
1															
2															
3															

Score	Description	Action

0 or 1	Awake and alert or Easy to rouse, stays awake for ≥10 seconds	• Check Sedation Score before administering opioids/potentially sedating medication
		• Check Sedation Score 1 hour post administering opioids/potentially sedating medication when it is:
		  » short acting; or
		  » a new medication; or
		  » an increased dose.

2	Easy to rouse but difficulty staying awake, falls asleep <10 seconds	• Ensure patient receives continuous oximetry monitoring and administer oxygen if oxygen saturations <94% • Withhold additional opioids/potentially sedating medication (until medical review) • Notify Team Leader • Notify Medical Officer who must review within 15 mins (remain with the patient until review) • Monitor CEWT and Sedation Score (minimum 15 minutely) until Sedation Score is less than 2 • If concerned, initiate **Emergency Call**
3	Difficult to rouse or unrousable	• Initiate **EMERGENCY CALL** • Ensure patient receives continuous oximetry monitoring and administer oxygen if oxygen saturations <94% • Administer naloxone as per order *(for opioids)* • Withhold additional opioids/potentially sedating medication • **Monitor CEWT and Sedation Score (minimum 5 minutely) until Sedation Score is less than 3**

Queensland Health Patient Safety and Quality, Clinical Excellence Queensland, Children's Early Warning Tool Version 3.0. © State of Queensland (Queensland Health) 2021

Figure 6.4, *continued*

DO NOT WRITE IN THIS BINDING MARGIN

pharmacological resources for doses and routes of administration of medications (International Association for the Study of Pain 2020).

Some common physiological indicators of pain that should be noted when assessing pain in children are:

- Increased heart rate (due to pain and anxiety)
- Respiratory rate changes (increase due to pain/anxiety/fear, decrease due to breath holding)
- Increase in blood pressure
- Oxygen saturation may decrease (paediatric patient may not want to breathe due to fear of pain).

There are three commonly used pain assessment tools used in paediatrics:

- Face, Legs, Activity, Cry and Consolability (FLACC)
- Wong–Baker Faces
- Visual Analogue Scale.

FLACC

The acronym FLACC stands for Face, Legs, Activity, Cry and Consolability. FLACC pain assessment tool (Fig. 6.5) is commonly used for children aged 2 months–8 years (can also be used for children aged up to 18 years). This tool is suitable for use with children with cognitive impairment and/or developmental

Category	Score		
	0	1	2
Face	No particular expression or smile	Occasional grimace or frown, withdrawn, disinterested	Frequent-to-constant quivering chin, clenched jaw
Legs	Normal position or relaxed	Uneasy, restless, tense	Kicking, or legs drawn up
Activity	Lying quietly, normal position, moves easily	Squirming, shifting back and forth, tense	Arched, rigid, or jerking
Cry	No cry (awake or asleep)	Moans or whimpers, occasional complaint	Crying steadily, screams or sobs, or frequent complaints
Consolability	Content, relaxed	Reassured by occasional touching, hugging, or being talked to, distractible	Difficult to console or comfort

Each of the five categories–(F) Face, (L) Legs, (A) Activity, (C) Cry, (C) Consolability–
is scored from 0-2, which results in a total score between 0 and 10.

Figure 6.5 FLACC Pain Assessment Tool. (Source: Workman and LaCharity 2016.)

Pain Scales Combined: NRS + FACES

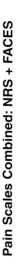
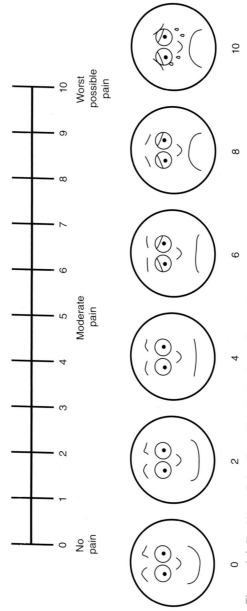

Figure 6.6 The Wong–Baker Faces Pain Rating Scale. (Source: From Hockenberry MJ, Wilson D, Rodgers CC. Wong's Essentials of Pediatric Nursing. 10th ed. St. Louis, MO: Elsevier; 2017:116.)

disability, with the involvement of their caregivers as assessment may be more difficult.

Wong–Baker Faces Pain Rating Scale

The Wong–Baker Faces Pain Rating Scale (Fig. 6.6) is commonly used for children 3–18 years old. The benefit of this tool is that patients themselves can indicate (by pointing to a picture) their pain levels.

Visual Analogue Scale

The Visual Analogue Scale (or Numeric Rating Scale) (Fig. 6.7) is commonly used on patients aged 8 years and older. If using the 'self-reporting' pain assessment tool, the patient needs to have a more advanced level of cognitive development.

> **Nursing alert**
>
> Always remember:
> * Assess pain using an appropriate pain assessment tool
> * Do not forget to REASSESS pain after interventions
> * Assess pain at rest and on movement
> * Document pain scores on CEWT
> * Use caregiver pain behavioural knowledge – they are the expert in the child's usual behaviour

Fluid balance charts

Fluid balance charts (Fig. 6.8) are important as part of assessment of a paediatric patient's fluid status. To accurately chart the

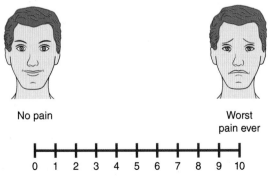

Figure 6.7 Visual Analogue Scale. (Source: Jennings 2024.)

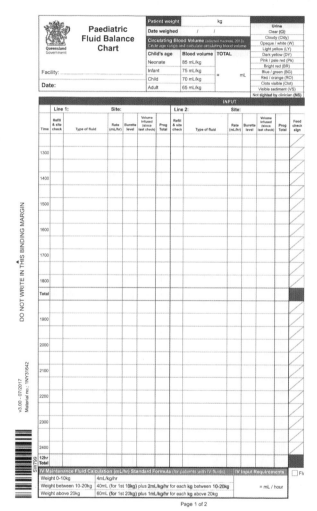

Figure 6.8 Fluid balance charts.

Description Code for Output

Vomit	Stool – colour	Drain / wound /other
Clear (Cl)	Brown (B)	Thin / watery (Tn)
Mixed food / milk (MF)	Yellow / orange (Y)	Thick (Tk)
Yellow (Y)	Green (G)	Clear (Cl)
Green (G)	White / clay / pale (W)	Opaque / white (W)
Brown / coffee (B)	Flecks / streaks red (FR)	Pink / pale red (Pk)
Dark red (DR)	Bright red (BR)	Bright red (BR)
Bright red (BR)	Dark Red (DR)	Tan / yellow (Y)
Clots visible (Clot)	Clots visible (Clot)	Brown (B)
Flecks / streaks red (FR)	Black (Blk)	Green (G)
Faecal odour (FO)	Offensive odour (OO)	Clots visible (Clot)
Not sighted by clinician (NS)	Not sighted by clinician (NS)	Offensive odour (OO)
	Refer Bristol Stool Chart for consistency	Not sighted by clinician (NS)

(Affix patient identification label here)

Oral/Enteral Intake					OUTPUT											Balance Summary			
					Urine			Stool		Vomit						In	Out	Balance	
Description	Oral volume	Tube volume	ng pH	Prog Total	Code	Volume	Prog total	ml/kg/hr	Code	Volume	Code	Volume	Code	Volume	Code	Volume			___ mLs POS / NEG	Time
																			1300
																			1400
																			1500
																			1600
																			1700
																			1800
																			Total
																			1900
																			2000
																			2100
																			2200
																			2300
																			2400
																			12hr Total

Fluid restriction:

_____ mLs / 24 hours

Expected Urine Output (mL/hr/kg) Standard Formula		Expected Urine Output	
Infant	• 2mL/kg/hr		
Child	• 1mL/kg/hr	= mL / hour	
Adolescent • 0.5-1mL/kg/hr			

☐ Fluid Balance Total escalated to Medical Officer

Time:

Paediatric Fluid Balance Chart

Queensland Government

Facility: _____

Date: _____

Patient weight		kg
Date weighed	/	/

Circulating Blood Volume (adapted Hazinski, 2013)
Circle age range and calculate circulating blood volume

Child's age	Blood volume	TOTAL		
Neonate	85 mL/kg			
Infant	75 mL/kg	=	mL	
Child	70 mL/kg			
Adult	65 mL/kg			

Description

Urine	Vomit
Clear (Cl)	Clear (Cl)
Cloudy (Cldy)	Mixed food / milk (MF)
Opaque / white (W)	Yellow (Y)
Light yellow (LY)	Green (G)
Dark yellow (DY)	Brown / coffee (B)
Pink / pale red (Pk)	Dark red (DR)
Bright red (BR)	Bright red (BR)
Blue / green (BG)	Clots visible (Clot)
Red / orange (RO)	Flecks / streaks red (FR)
Clots visible (Clot)	Faecal odour (FO)
Visible sediment (VS)	Not sighted by clinician (NS)
Not sighted by clinician (NS)	

INPUT

Time	Line 1: Refill & site check	Type of fluid	Rate (mL/hr)	Burette level	Volume infused (since last check)	Prog Total	Line 2: Refill & site check	Type of fluid	Rate (mL/hr)	Burette level	Volume infused (since last check)	Prog Total	Feed check sign	Oral/Enteral Description
Prev. total														
0100														
0200														
0300														
0400														
0500														
0600														
Total														
0700														
0800														
0900														
1000														
1100														
1200														
24hr Total														

Line 1: Site: ___   Line 2: Site: ___

IV Maintenance Fluid Calculation (mL/hr) Standard Formula (for patients with IV fluids)

Weight 0-10kg	4mL/kg/hr
Weight between 10-20kg	40mL (for 1st 10kg) plus 2mL/kg/hr for each kg between 10-20kg
Weight above 20kg	60mL (for 1st 20kg) plus 1mL/kg/hr for each kg above 20kg

IV Input Requirements = mL / hour

☐ Fluid restriction: _____ mLs / 24

Figure 6.8, *continued*

Code for Output

Stool – colour	Drain / wound /other
Brown (B)	Thin / watery (Tn)
Yellow / orange (Y)	Thick (Tk)
Green (G)	Clear (Cl)
White / clay / pale (W)	Opaque / white (W)
Flecks / streaks red (FR)	Pink / pale red (Pk)
Bright red (BR)	Bright red (BR)
Dark Red (DR)	Tan / yellow (Y)
Clots visible (Clot)	Brown (B)
Black (Blk)	Green (G)
Offensive odour (OO)	Clots visible (Clot)
Not sighted by clinician (NS)	Offensive odour (OO)
Refer Bristol Stool Chart for consistency	Not sighted by clinician (NS)

(Affix patient identification label here)

Intake				OUTPUT												Balance Summary			
				Urine				Stool		Vomit						In	Out	Balance	
Oral volume	Tube volume	ng pH	Prog Total	Code	Volume	Prog total	ml/kg/hr	Code	Volume	Code	Volume	Code	Volume	Code	Volume			.... mLs POS / NEG	Time
																			Prev. total
																			0100
																			0200
																			0300
																			0400
																			0500
																			0600
																			Total
																			0700
																			0800
																			0900
																			1000
																			1100
																			1200
																			24hr Total

hours

Expected Urine Output (mL/hr/kg) Standard Formula	Expected Urine Output
Infant ▸ 2mL/kg/hr	
Child ▸ 1mL/kg/hr	= mL / hour
Adolescent ▸ 0.5-1mL/kg/hr	

☐ Fluid Balance Total escalated to Medical Officer
Time: ....

DO NOT WRITE IN THIS BINDING MARGIN

paediatric patient's fluid balance, nurses are expected to calculate several components based on the weight of the paediatric patient. The fluid balance requires the following calculations:

- Circulating blood volume
- IV maintenance fluid calculation
- Expected urine output.

Nurses are expected to calculate fluid input and output and make a clinical decision about the paediatric patient's fluid status and act in response to that.

To assist the nurse with an assessment of a paediatric patient, a rapid assessment known as the Paediatric Assessment Triangle (Horeczko et al 2013; Fig. 6.9) can be utilised to assess an unwell child quickly and efficiently to determine if immediate intervention is required. Focusing on appearance, breathing and circulation, it provides a first impression of the sick child:

- Appearance – observe tone, intractability, consolability, look or gaze and speech or cry
- Breathing – observe for nasal flaring, retractions, abnormal airway sounds, position of comfort, altered respiratory rate
- Circulation to skin – observe for pallor, mottling cyanosis.

Also, see Figure 6.10 for tips for shift changeover with medications and IV fluids.

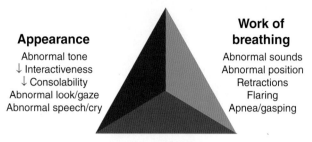

Figure 6.9 The Pediatric Assessment Triangle and its components.
(Horeczko et al 2013.)

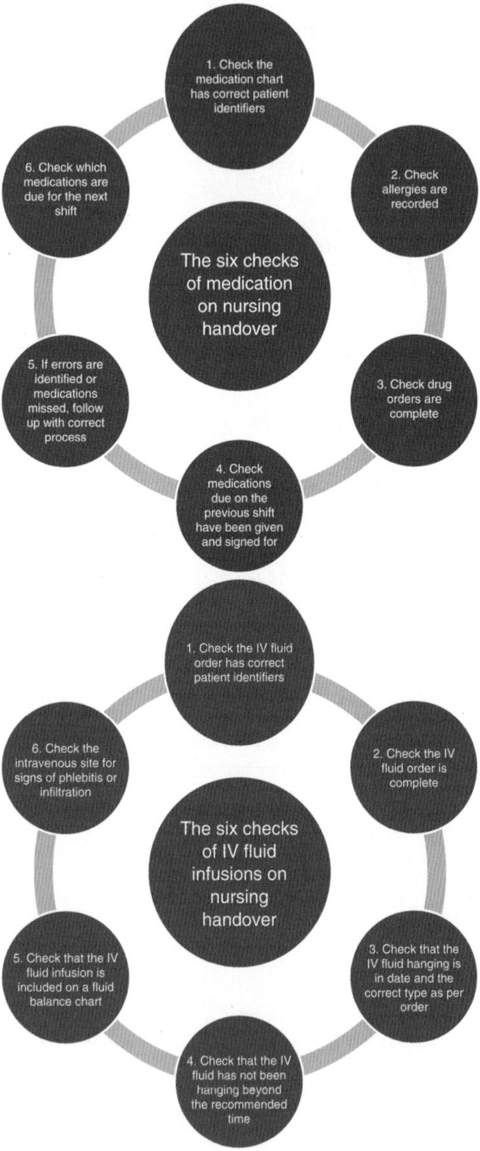

The six checks of medication on nursing handover

1. Check the medication chart has correct patient identifiers
2. Check allergies are recorded
3. Check drug orders are complete
4. Check medications due on the previous shift have been given and signed for
5. If errors are identified or medications missed, follow up with correct process
6. Check which medications are due for the next shift

The six checks of IV fluid infusions on nursing handover

1. Check the IV fluid order has correct patient identifiers
2. Check the IV fluid order is complete
3. Check that the IV fluid hanging is in date and the correct type as per order
4. Check that the IV fluid has not been hanging beyond the recommended time
5. Check that the IV fluid infusion is included on a fluid balance chart
6. Check the intravenous site for signs of phlebitis or infiltration

Figure 6.10 Tips for shift changeover with medications and/or intravenous fluids.

Skill audits

Rinnah Peacock, Kerry Reid-Searl,
Pauline Davies

Paediatric skill 7.1
ADMINISTERING ENTERAL FEEDING VIA NASOGASTRIC TUBE (NGT)

This task must be undertaken by an appropriately qualified nurse and therefore cannot be delegated to untrained clinicians (e.g., AINs, students). Untrained clinicians must be supervised if completing skills as part of training or upskilling.

Special considerations
- Confirm paediatric patient's identity.
- Gain consent from both the paediatric patient and caregiver.
- Build rapport with the paediatric patient and caregiver.
- Explain procedure to the paediatric patient and caregiver in a manner that is appropriate for their learning styles and ages.
- Discuss procedure with the paediatric patient (invest time into this as the paediatric patient may want to perform the procedure on a mannequin/puppet or watch a video on procedure to gain more understanding, etc.).
- Be honest about actions and potential discomfort at all stages of procedure.
- Provide reassurance and use distraction methods, if appropriate.
- Ensure the medication has been ordered for the right reason.
- Check medication information using appropriate resources; for example, paediatric injectables book, including compatibility

with other prescribed medications. If contraindications exist, withhold medication and inform prescriber.

- Review data that may influence medication administration.
- Review physical examination and laboratory data that may influence medication administration.

Equipment

- Disposable feeding bag and tubing or ready-to-hang system
- 30 mL or larger ENFit syringe
- Stethoscope
- pH indicator strip
- Infusion pump (required for intestinal feedings): use pump designed for tube feedings
- Prescribed enteral feedings
- Gloves
- Equipment to obtain blood glucose by finger-stick
- Paediatric National Inpatient Medication Chart (NIMC) or equivalent electronic record.

Assess the paediatric patient's need for enteral tube feedings:
- Impaired swallowing/sucking
- Decreased level of consciousness
- Head or neck surgery, facial trauma
- Surgeries of upper alimentary canal
- Unable to consume adequate nutrition
- Facial or esophageal structural abnormalities
- Eating disorders
- Congenital anomalies
- Primary disease management

Auscultate for bowel sounds before feeding

Obtain baseline weight and laboratory values. Assess the paediatric patient for fluid volume excess or deficit, electrolyte abnormalities and metabolic abnormalities such as hyperglycemia

Verify the order for formula, rate, route and frequency. Laboratory data and bedside assessments, such as finger-stick blood glucose measurement, may also be required

Explain procedure to the paediatric patient and caregiver

Wash hands

Prepare feeding container to administer formula:
- Have tube feeding at room temperature
- Connect tubing to container as needed or prepare ready-to-hang container

If a ready-to-hang container is not available, shake formula container well, and fill feeding bag and tubing with formula

Place the paediatric patient in high-Fowler's position or elevate head of bed 30 degrees. When preparing to administer feeds, nursing staff should again check the tube's position and flush it before and after the feed

Determine tube placement: this should occur prior to each feed, before each medication, before putting anything down the tube, if the paediatric patient has vomited and fourth-hourly for continuous feeds

- Don personal protective equipment (PPE) – gloves
- Use an enteral/oral syringe (10–20 mL for an infant/child or a 5–10 mL for a neonate) and attach to the enteral tube
- Aspirate minimum 0.5–1 mL of gastric content (sufficient to enable pH testing). Consider the 'dead space' in the tubing. Using pH indicator strips a reading of between 0–5 should be obtained and documented
- Observe the aspirate's appearance
- Consider the results from pH testing, the aspirate's appearance and compare the insertion length of the feeding tube to what was originally verified on insertion

Critical decision point: auscultation is no longer considered a reliable method for verification of placement of tube because air in tube inadvertently placed in lungs, pharynx or oesophagus can transmit sound similar to that of air entering stomach

Initiate feeding
Points to remember once paediatric NGT feeds are commenced:
a. The following needs to be checked second-hourly during feeds:
   - Taping
   - Marker on the NGT
   - Signs of respiratory distress
b. Check infusion hourly and document intake
c. Feeds should hang for no longer than 4 hours to reduce the risk of bacterial growth

Bolus or intermittent feeding
Using a syringe for a bolus feed:
- Remove the plunger from the syringe and place the tip of the syringe into the enteral tube connector at the end of the enteral tube
- Hold the syringe and connected enteral tube upright and pour the required fluid into the syringe. The flow rate should be slow – the rate can be adjusted by the height the syringe is held as it flows via gravity
- At completion, follow through with the prescribed water to flush the feed through the tubing

Continuous-drip method
- Hang feeding bag and tubing on a pole
- Connect the distal end of tubing to the proximal end of the feeding tube
- Connect tubing through infusion pump and set rate

Advance tube feeding as recommended by the dietitian or doctor

When feeding is complete, flush the tubing with the prescribed amount of water. Chart the amount of water on the fluid balance chart

When tube feedings are not being administered, cap or clamp the proximal end of the feeding tube

Administer water via feeding tube as ordered with diluted formula

Rinse bag and tubing with warm water whenever feedings are interrupted for prolonged periods. Follow the manufacturer's recommendations as some feeding bags are recommended as single use only

Measure the amount of aspirate (residual) every 4–6 hours, if required

Monitor intake and output every 24 hours

Weigh the paediatric patient weekly after admission unless otherwise indicated

Documentation
- Record administration of medication on paediatric NIMIC and add both nurses' initials, signature or appropriate electronic identifier
- Record amount and type of feeding
- Record the paediatric patient's response to tube feeding, patency of tube
- Report tolerance and adverse effects

(Adapted from Rebeiro et al 2021.)

Paediatric skill 7.2

ADDING MEDICATIONS TO INTRAVENOUS FLUID CONTAINERS

This task must be undertaken by an appropriately qualified nurse and therefore cannot be delegated to untrained clinicians (e.g., AINs, students). Untrained clinicians must be supervised if completing skills as part of training or upskilling.

Special considerations
- Confirm paediatric patient's identity.
- Gain consent from both the paediatric patient and caregiver.
- Build rapport with patient and caregiver.
- Explain procedure to the paediatric patient and caregiver in a manner that is appropriate for their learning styles and ages.

- Discuss procedure with the paediatric patient (invest time into this as the paediatric patient may want to perform procedure on a mannequin/puppet or watch a video on procedure to gain more understanding etc.).
- Be honest about actions and potential discomfort at all stages of procedure.
- Provide reassurance and use distraction methods, if appropriate.
- Ensure the medication has been ordered for the right reason.
- Check medication information using appropriate resources; for example, paediatric injectables book, including compatibility with other prescribed medications. If contraindications exist, withhold medication and inform prescriber.
- Review data that may influence medication administration.
- Review physical examination and laboratory data that may influence medication administration.

Equipment
- Appropriate PPE (non-sterile gloves)
- Vial or ampoule of prescribed medication
- Syringe of appropriate size (5–20 mL)
- Sterile vial access cannula or drawing-up needle (18–21 gauge) or blunt filter drawing-up needle
- Correct diluent (e.g., sterile water, 0.9% sodium chloride)
- Sterile IV fluid container of ordered fluid volume
- Alcohol or antiseptic swab
- Additive label to attach to IV bag or bottle
- Paediatric NIMC or equivalent electronic record.

Identify the prescription order contains all essential elements: prescriber details, paediatric patient details, medication name, medication dose, medication route, frequency of medication administration

Ensure weight of the paediatric patient is recorded

Ensure the dose ordered is appropriate for the weight and age of the paediatric patient

Assess the paediatric patient for allergies and/or sensitivities and check medication alerts. Check with caregiver

Ensure the medication has been ordered for the right reason. If this is not apparent, the appropriately qualified nurse should contact the prescriber

Collect information necessary to administer drug safely, including action, purpose, side effects, dose is weight/age appropriate, time of peak onset and nursing implications

Perform hand hygiene and use gloves if this is agency policy (i.e., for cytotoxic or antibiotic medicines)

Assemble supplies in medication room (or other area as designated by clinical agency). Ensure correct number of persons present for preparing medication. This includes an appropriately qualified nurse and another medication endorsed nurse

Perform first medication check:
- Right patient
- Right medication
- Right dose
- Right route
- Right time/frequency
- Right documentation

Prepare prescribed medication from vial or ampoule

Perform second medication check and Independent Second Check by another appropriately qualified nurse
- Right patient
- Right medication
- Right dose
- Right route
- Right time/frequency
- Right documentation

Add medication to new container

Solution in a bag:
- Locate medication injection port on plastic IV solution bag. Port has small stopper at end. Do not select port for the IV tubing insertion or air vent

Solution in a bottle:
- Locate injection site on IV solution bottle, which is often covered by a cap

Solution in a burette:
- Locate the injection site on the top of the burette. Do not select port for the IV connection to the bag of fluid above

Wipe port or injection site with alcohol/antiseptic swab

Remove needle cap or sheath from syringe and insert needle of syringe or needleless device through centre of injection port or site; inject medication

If inserting medication into a burette, it may be necessary to administer a small flush of normal saline to clear any residual medication from the access site

Withdraw syringe from bag, bottle or burette

Mix medication and IV solution by holding bag or bottle and turning it gently end to end. For a burette, do not invert, simply hold, and gently swirl the burette

Complete medication label with name and dose of medication, date, time and both nurses' initials and attach to bottle, bag or burette

Spike bag or bottle with IV tubing and prime the tubing with the fluid

Administer medication
- Perform hand hygiene
- Proceed to patient with medication
- Perform third medication check:
  - Right patient
  - Right medication
  - Right dose according to weight and age
  - Right route
  - Right time/frequency
  - Right documentation
- Prepare paediatric patient and caregiver
  - Explain that medication is to be given through existing IV line or one to be started
  - Explain that in general discomfort may be felt during medication infusion; however, depending on the rate of the infusion, coolness can be felt at the site
  - Encourage paediatric patient and caregiver to report symptoms of discomfort, including pain and swelling
- Monitor the paediatric patient and site regularly throughout the infusion

Set up the infusion in the volumetric infusion pump using the required guard rails. Regulate infusion at prescribed rate

Perform hand hygiene

Regularly assess:
- IV cannula insertion site
- Rate of infusion
- Signs of adverse reaction
- Fluid volume excess

Documentation
- Record administration of medication on paediatric NIMIC and add both nurses' initials, signature or appropriate electronic identifier
- Report any adverse reactions to an appropriately qualified nurse in charge or prescriber

(Adapted from Rebeiro et al 2021.)

Paediatric skill 7.3

ADMINISTERING ORAL MEDICATIONS

This task must be undertaken by an appropriately qualified nurse and therefore cannot be delegated to untrained clinicians (e.g., AINs, students). Untrained clinicians must be supervised if completing skills as part of training or upskilling.

Special considerations

- Confirm paediatric patient's identity.
- Gain consent from both the paediatric patient and caregiver.
- Build rapport with patient and caregiver.
- Explain procedure to the paediatric patient and caregiver in a manner that is appropriate for their learning styles and ages.
- Discuss procedure with the paediatric patient (invest time into this as paediatric patient may want to perform procedure on a mannequin/puppet or watch a video on procedure to gain more understanding, etc.).
- Be honest about actions and potential discomfort at all stages of procedure.
- Provide reassurance and use distraction methods, if appropriate.
- Ensure the medication has been ordered for the right reason.
- Check medication information using appropriate resources including compatibility with other prescribed medications. If contraindications exist, withhold medication and inform prescriber.
- Review data that may influence medication administration.
- Review physical examination and laboratory data that may influence medication administration.

Equipment

- Medication trolley/pharmacy on wheels (if applicable).
- Disposable medication cups.
- Glass of water, juice or preferred liquid.
- Clean pill-crusher (if required).
- Paediatric NIMC or equivalent electronic record.

Identify that the prescription order contains all essential elements: prescriber details, patient details, medication name, medication dose, medication route, frequency of medication administration

Assess the paediatric patient for allergies and/or sensitivities and check medication alerts

Ensure the medication has been ordered for the right reason. If this is not apparent, an appropriately qualified nurse should contact the prescriber

Assess the suitability of administration via the oral route

- Is the paediatric patient suffering from nausea/vomiting?

Check the paediatric patient's swallow, cough and gag reflexes have been assessed, if in doubt about patient's ability to manage oral medications

Withhold medication if swallow, cough or gag is impaired and notify prescriber

If the paediatric patient has difficulty swallowing, ask the prescriber to substitute with liquid or dissolvable preparation. If liquid medications are not an option, use a clean pill-crushing device such as a mortar and pestle to grind tablets. Always check that the medication can be crushed

- Mix ground tablet in small amount of soft food
  OR
- Dissolve in water to form a liquid that can be swallowed
  Assess the paediatric patient's preferences for fluids

Prepare medication

- Perform hand hygiene
- Select correct medication
- Check expiration date on all medications
- Calculate medication dose, as necessary. Double-check calculation

  Perform first medication check:
- Right patient
- Right medication
- Right dose
- Right route
- Right time/frequency
- Right documentation

  Prepare medication appropriately

  Perform second medication check and Independent Second Check by another appropriately qualified nurse:
- Right patient
- Right medication
- Right dose
- Right route
- Right time/frequency
- Right documentation

  Proceed to paediatric patient with medication at correct time
  Perform third medication check:
- Ask patient to state name and date of birth while verifying ID band, and then comparing against paediatric NIMC
- Right medication
- Right dose
- Right route
- Right time (and frequency)
- Right documentation

  Explain purpose of each medication and its action to paediatric patient. Allow the patient to ask any questions about medication. This needs to be age-appropriate explanations for both patient and caregiver

Assist paediatric patient to an appropriate position. Help the
patient to sit or to lie on the side if sitting is contraindicated
Offer water or juice to help patients swallow medications

Sublingually administered medications
Have patients place medication under their tongue and allow it to
dissolve completely. Caution the patient against swallowing tablets.
Distraction is often required to take the focus away from swallowing
the tablet

Buccally administered medication
Have the patient place medication in the mouth against mucous
membranes of the cheek until it dissolves. Avoid administering liquids
until buccal medication has dissolved
Mix powdered medications with liquids at bedside and give to
patient to drink. This may need to be completed in medication room
as can heighten anxiety for the paediatric patient. Either way, quick
administration of medication assists to ensure medication does not
become cloggy
Give effervescent powders and tablets immediately after dissolving
Stay until the patient has completely swallowed each medication
Perform hand hygiene
Return within 30 min to evaluate patient's response to medications
Always notify the prescriber when the patient exhibits an adverse
effect or allergic reaction

Documentation
- Record administration of medication on paediatric NIMIC and
  add both nurses' initials, signature or appropriate electronic
  identifier
- Report tolerance and adverse effects

(Adapted from Rebeiro et al 2021; Educational Resource Centre, Women's &
Children's Health, 2001. How to give medications to children. Available at: https://
www.rch.org.au/uploadedFiles/Main/Content/pharmacy/how-to-give-medications-
to-children.pdf.)

Paediatric skill 7.4
ADMINISTERING RECTAL SUPPOSITORIES

This task must be undertaken by an appropriately qualified nurse
and therefore cannot be delegated to untrained clinicians (e.g.,
AINs, students). Untrained clinicians must be supervised if completing the skill as part of training or upskilling.

Special considerations
- Confirm paediatric patient's identity.

- Gain consent from both the paediatric patient and caregiver.
- Build rapport with patient and caregiver.
- Explain procedure to the paediatric patient and caregiver in a manner that is appropriate for their learning styles and ages.
- Discuss procedure with the paediatric patient (invest time into this as paediatric patient may want to perform procedure on a mannequin/puppet or watch a video on procedure to gain more understanding, etc.).
- Be honest about actions and potential discomfort at all stages of procedure.
- Provide reassurance and use distraction methods, if appropriate.
- Ensure the medication has been ordered for the right reason.
- Check medication information using appropriate resources including compatibility with other prescribed medications. If contraindications exist, withhold medication and inform prescriber.
- Review data that may influence medication administration.
- Review physical examination and laboratory data that may influence medication administration.

Equipment
- Rectal suppository
- Lubricating jelly (water-soluble)
- Disposable gloves
- Tissue
- Drape
- Paediatric National Inpatient Medication Chart (NIMC) or equivalent electronic record.

Identify the prescription order contains all essential elements: prescriber details, patient details, medication name, medication dose, medication route, frequency of medication administration
   Assess patient for allergies and/or sensitivities and check medication alerts
   Ensure the medication has been ordered for the right reason. If this is not apparent, an appropriately qualified nurse should contact the prescriber
   Assess for suitability of administration via the rectal route
   Is patient experiencing rectal bleeding?

Prepare medication
- Perform hand hygiene
- Select correct medication
- Check expiration date on all medications
  Perform first medication check:
- Right patient
- Right medication
- Right dose
- Right route
- Right time/frequency
- Right documentation
  Ensures patient understands procedure
  Perform second medication check and Independent Second
Check by another appropriately qualified nurse:
- Right patient
- Right medication
- Right dose
- Right route
- Right time/frequency
- Right documentation
  Proceed to the patient with the medication at correct time
  Perform third medication check:
- Right patient
- Right medication
- Right dose
- Right route
- Right time/frequency
- Right documentation
  Close door or curtain
  Perform hand hygiene
  Position patient on left side with upper leg bent and buttocks
separated
  Put on disposable gloves
  Remove suppository from wrapper and lubricate rounded end to
be inserted initially
  Ask patient to take slow deep breaths through mouth or
distraction method discussed in preparation process
  Retract buttocks with non-dominant hand. Insert suppository
gently through anus:
- for bullet-shaped suppository, insert the smooth, pointy end first
- for tear-shaped suppository, insert the larger, rounded end first
  Hold the buttocks together for 5 min. Distraction will be needed
for this
  Withdraw finger and wipe anal area with tissue
  Discard gloves and dispose of them in appropriate receptacle
  Ask patient to lie down or sit down for about 10 min. Distraction
techniques will be of assistance for this duration
  If suppository contains laxative or faecal softener, place call light
within reach

Perform hand hygiene
Observe for effects of suppository (e.g., bowel movement, relief of nausea) 30 min after administration

Documentation
- Record administration of medication on paediatric NIMIC and add both appropriately qualified nurses' initials, signature or appropriate electronic identifier
- Report tolerance and adverse effects

(Adapted from Rebeiro et al 2021; Educational Resource Centre, Women's & Children's Health, 2001. How to give medications to children. Available at: https://www.rch.org.au/uploadedFiles/Main/Content/pharmacy/how-to-give-medications-to-children.pdf.)

Paediatric skill 7.5

ADMINISTERING METERED-DOSE INHALERS (MDIS)

This task must be undertaken by an appropriately qualified nurse and therefore cannot be delegated to untrained clinicians (e.g., AINs, students). Untrained clinicians must be supervised if completing the skill as part of training or upskilling.

Special considerations
- Confirm paediatric patient's identity.
- Gain consent from both the paediatric patient and caregiver.
- Build rapport with patient and caregiver.
- Explain procedure to paediatric patient and caregiver in a manner that is appropriate for their learning styles and ages.
- Discuss procedure with the paediatric patient (invest time into this as the paediatric patient may want to perform procedure on a mannequin/puppet or watch a video on procedure to gain more understanding, etc.).
- Be honest about actions and potential discomfort at all stages of procedure.
- Provide reassurance and use distraction methods, if appropriate.
- Ensure the medication has been ordered for the right reason.
- Check medication information using appropriate resources; for example, APMH, including compatibility with other

prescribed medications. If contraindications exist, withhold medication and inform prescriber.

- Review data that may influence medication administration.
- Review physical examination and laboratory data that may influence medication administration.

Equipment

- MDI with medication canister
- Spacer (e.g., volumatic) – optional
- Facial tissues – optional
- Paper towel
- Paediatric NIMC or equivalent electronic record.

Identify that the prescription order contains all essential elements: prescriber details, patient details, medication name, medication dose, medication route, frequency of medication administration
  Assess patient for allergies and/or sensitivities and check medication alerts
  Assess for suitability of administration via the inhalation route
  Assess paediatric patient's ability to self-administer inhaler. The paediatric patient often requires assistance with:
  – Holding the MDI in mouth and depressing canister
  – Sealing the MDI with mouth (if this cannot be achieved, a mask can be used)
  Assess patient's readiness and ability to learn and understand the procedure
  If previously instructed in self-administration of inhaled medicine, assess patient's/caregiver's technique in using an inhaler
  Instruct patient in comfortable environment
  Perform first medication check:
- Right patient
- Right medication
- Right dose
- Right route
- Right time/frequency
- Right documentation

Prepare medication
- Perform hand hygiene and arrange equipment needed
- Select correct medication
  Perform second medication check and Independent Second Check by another an appropriately qualified nurse:
- Right patient
- Right medication
- Right dose
- Right route
- Right time/frequency
- Right documentation

Allow patient opportunity to manipulate inhaler, canister and spacer device. Explain and demonstrate how canister fits into inhaler

Explain what metered dose is, and warn about overuse of inhaler, including medication side effects

Perform third medication check:

- Right patient
- Right medication
- Right dose
- Right route
- Right time/frequency
- Right documentation

Explain steps for administering inhaled dose of medication (demonstrate steps when possible)

When using a spacer or mask with MDI:

- Insert MDI into end of spacer
- Shake inhaler well
- Prime a brand-new spacer before use (with 10 puffs of salbutamol)
- Place spacer mouthpiece in mouth and close lips
- Do not insert beyond raised lip on mouthpiece
- Avoid covering small exhalation slots with the lips
- Breathe normally through spacer mouthpiece
- Depress medication canister, spraying one puff into spacer
- Ask patient to breathe in and out normally for four breaths

Shake the puffer and spacer between each dose until number of doses ordered is administered

Explain that patient may feel gagging sensation in throat caused by droplets of medication on pharynx or tongue

Instruct patient to rinse mouth or have a drink of water

Instruct patient in removing medication canister and cleaning inhaler in warm water

Ask if patient/caregiver has any questions

After medication instillation, assess patient's respirations and auscultate lungs

Documentation

- Record administration of medication on paediatric NIMIC and add both appropriately qualified nurses' initials, signature or appropriate electronic identifier
- Report tolerance and adverse effects

(Adapted from Rebeiro et al 2021, Children's Health Queensland Hospital and Health Service 2022 Puffers and spacers. Available at: https://www.childrens. health.qld.gov.au/health-a-to-z/puffers-and-spacers; Children's Health Queensland Hospital and Health Service Asthma – Emergency guideline. Available at: https:// www.childrens.health.qld.gov.au/for-health-professionals/queensland-paediatric-emergency-care-qpec/queensland-paediatric-clinical-guidelines/asthma, National Asthma Council Australia. Available at: https://www.nationalasthma.org.au/.)

Paediatric skill 7.6

PREPARING INJECTIONS

This task must be undertaken by an appropriately qualified nurse and therefore cannot be delegated to untrained clinicians (e.g., AINs, students). Untrained clinicians must be supervised if completing skills as part of training or upskilling.

Special considerations

- Confirm paediatric patient's identity.
- Gain consent from both the paediatric patient and caregiver.
- Build rapport with patient and caregiver.
- Explain procedure to paediatric patient and caregiver in a manner that is appropriate for their learning styles and ages.
- Discuss procedure with the paediatric patient (invest time into this as paediatric patient may want to perform the procedure on a mannequin/puppet or watch a video on procedure to gain more understanding, etc.).
- Be honest about actions and potential discomfort at all stages of procedure.
- Provide reassurance and use distraction methods, if appropriate.
- Ensure the medication has been ordered for the right reason.
- Check medication information using appropriate resources; for example, paediatric injectables book, including compatibility with other prescribed medications. If contraindications exist, withhold medication and inform prescriber.
- Review data that may influence medication administration.
- Review physical examination and laboratory data that may influence medication administration.

Equipment

- Correct size syringe and needle:
  - Drawing-up needles (18-gauge blunt needle) or vial access cannula (intravenous) or blunt filter needles for glass ampoules
  - Subcutaneous (sub cut): syringe (1–3 mL) and needle (25–30 gauge)
  - Intramuscular (IM): syringe 2–3 mL for adults, 0.5–1 mL for infants and small children. Two needles: 21–24 gauge

   – Intradermal (ID): 1 mL tuberculin syringe with pre-attached 26- or 27-gauge needle
- Small gauze pad and/or alcohol swab
- Vial or ampoule of medication or skin test solution
- Disposable gloves.

Additional equipment
- Medication in an ampoule:
   – Small gauze pad or alcohol swab
- Medication in a vial:
   – Small gauze pad or alcohol swab
   – Compatible diluent (e.g., 0.0% sodium chloride or sterile water)
- Paediatric NIMC or equivalent electronic record.

Tap the top of ampoule lightly and quickly with your finger until fluid moves from neck of ampoule
   Place a small gauze pad around neck of ampoule
   Snap neck of ampoule quickly and firmly away from hands
   Hold the ampoule upside down or set it on a flat surface. Insert the drawing-up needle into centre of ampoule opening. Do not allow blunt filter needle tip or shaft to touch rim of ampoule
- Aspirate medication into syringe by gently pulling back on plunger
- Keep blunt filter needle tip under surface of liquid. Tip ampoule to bring all fluid within reach of the needle
   To expel excess air bubbles, remove needle from ampoule. Hold syringe with needle pointing up. Tap side of syringe to cause bubbles to rise towards needle. Draw back slightly on plunger, and then push plunger upwards to eject air. Do not eject medication
   If syringe contains excess medication, dispose of appropriately. Recheck medication level in syringe by holding it vertically
   Change needle on syringe

Vial containing a solution
- Remove cap covering top of unused vial to expose sterile rubber seal, keeping rubber seal sterile. If reusing multi-dose vial, firmly and briskly wipe surface of rubber seal with alcohol swab and allow it to dry
- Pick up syringe and remove cap of needle or vial access cannula. Pull back on plunger to draw amount of air into syringe equivalent to volume of medication to be aspirated from vial

- With vial on flat surface, insert tip of needle/vial access cannula with bevelled tip entering first through centre of rubber seal
- Inject air into the vial's airspace, holding on to plunger. Hold plunger with firm pressure; plunger may be forced backwards by air pressure within the vial
- Invert vial while keeping firm hold on syringe and plunger. Hold vial between thumb and middle fingers of non-dominant hand. Grasp the end of syringe barrel and plunger with the thumb and forefinger of the dominant hand to counteract pressure in the vial
- Keep tip of needle/vial access cannula below fluid level
- Allow air pressure from the vial to fill syringe gradually with medication. If necessary, pull back slightly on plunger to obtain correct amount of solution
- When desired volume has been obtained, position needle/vial access cannula into vial's airspace; tap side of syringe barrel carefully to dislodge any air bubbles. Eject any air remaining at top of syringe into vial
- Remove needle/vial access cannula from vial by pulling back on barrel of syringe
- Hold the syringe at eye level, at a 90-degree angle, to ensure correct volume and absence of air bubbles. Remove any remaining air by tapping barrel to dislodge any air bubbles. Draw back slightly on plunger; then push plunger upwards to eject air. Do not eject fluid
- Remove vial access cannula/needle. Change to appropriate needle gauge and length if required according to route of medication

Vial containing a powder (reconstituting medications)
- Remove cap covering vial of powdered medication. Wipe rubber seal with alcohol wipe
- Draw up diluent into syringe
- Insert tip of needle/vial access cannula through centre of rubber seal of vial of powdered medication. Inject diluent into vial. Remove needle
- Mix medication thoroughly. Roll in palms. Do not shake
- Calculate dose using standard formula. (See Basic formulae for calculation of drug doses in Ch 1)
- Draw up the prescribed volume of reconstituted medication into syringe
- Dispose of soiled supplies. Place broken ampoule and/or used vials and used needle in puncture-proof and leak-proof sharps container. Clean work area and perform hand hygiene
- Keep tip of needle/vial access cannula below fluid level
- Allow air pressure from the vial to fill syringe gradually with medication. If necessary, pull back slightly on plunger to obtain correct amount of solution

- When desired volume has been obtained, position needle/vial access cannula into vial's airspace; tap side of syringe barrel carefully to dislodge any air bubbles. Eject any air remaining at top of syringe into vial
- Remove needle/vial access cannula from vial by pulling back on barrel of syringe
- Hold the syringe at eye level, at a 90-degree angle, to ensure correct volume and absence of air bubbles. Remove any remaining air by tapping barrel to dislodge any air bubbles. Draw back slightly on plunger; then push plunger upwards to eject air. Do not eject fluid
- Remove vial access cannula/needle. Change to appropriate needle gauge and length if required according to route of medication

(Adapted from Rebeiro et al 2021.)

Paediatric skill 7.7

ADMINISTERING INJECTIONS

This task must be undertaken by an appropriately qualified nurse and therefore cannot be delegated to untrained clinicians (e.g., AINs, students). Untrained clinicians must be supervised if completing skills as part of training or upskilling.

Special considerations

- Confirm paediatric patient's identity.
- Gain consent from both the paediatric patient and caregiver.
- Build rapport with patient and caregiver.
- Explain procedure to the paediatric patient and caregiver in a manner that is appropriate for their learning styles and ages.
- Discuss procedure with the paediatric patient (invest time into this as the paediatric patient may want to perform procedure on a mannequin/puppet or watch a video on procedure to gain more understanding, etc.).
- Be honest about actions and potential discomfort at all stages of procedure.
- Provide reassurance and use distraction methods, if appropriate.
- Ensure the medication has been ordered for the right reason.
- Check medication information using appropriate resources; for example, paediatrics injectables book, including compatibility

with other prescribed medications. If contraindications exist, withhold medication and inform prescriber.

- Review data that may influence medication administration.
- Review physical examination and laboratory data that may influence medication administration.

Equipment

- Correct size syringe and needle:
  - Drawing-up needles (18-gauge blunt needle) or vial access cannula (IV) or blunt filter needles for glass ampoules
  - Subcutaneous (sub cut): syringe (1–3 mL) and needle (25–30 gauge)
  - Intramuscular (IM): syringe 2–3 mL for adults, 0.5–1 mL for infants and small children. Two needles: 21–24 gauge
  - Intradermal (ID): 1 mL tuberculin syringe with pre-attached 26- or 27-gauge needle
- Small gauze pad and/or alcohol swab
- Vial or ampoule of medication or skin test solution
- Disposable gloves
- Paediatric NIMC or equivalent electronic record.

Identify the prescription order contains all essential elements: prescriber details, patient details, medication name, medication dose, medication route, frequency of medication administration

Assess patient for allergies and/or sensitivities and check medication alerts

Ensure the medication has been ordered for the right reason. If this is not apparent, an appropriately qualified nurse should contact the prescriber

Assess for suitability of administration via the injectable route and assess for contraindications

- Check resource material (e.g., *MIMS*, *AMH*, *PIG* [Lilley et al 2019], *Australian Injectable Drugs Handbook*)

Comparison of angles of insertion for intramuscular (90 degrees), subcutaneous (45 degrees) and intradermal (15 degrees) injections

For subcutaneous injections
Assess for factors such as circulatory shock or reduced local tissue perfusion. Assess adequacy of patient's adipose tissue

For intramuscular injections
Assess for factors such as muscle atrophy, reduced blood flow or circulatory shock

Prepare medication

Select correct medication. Compare label of medication with paediatric NIMC

Check expiration date on all medications

Perform first medication check:

- Right patient
- Right medication
- Right dose
- Right route
- Right time/frequency
- Right documentation

Calculate medication dose, as necessary. Double-check calculation

Perform hand hygiene

Prepare correct medication dose from ampoule or vial. Check carefully. Be sure all air is expelled

Perform second medication check and Independent Second Check by another appropriately qualified nurse:

- Right patient
- Right medication
- Right dose
- Right route
- Right time/frequency
- Right documentation

Proceed to patient with medication at correct time

Close room curtain or door

Explain steps of procedure and tell patient injection will cause a slight burning or sting

Perform first medication check:

- Right patient
- Right medication
- Right dose
- Right route
- Right time/frequency
- Right documentation

Perform hand hygiene; apply disposable gloves

Keep sheet or gown draped over body parts not requiring exposure

Select appropriate injection site. Inspect skin surface over sites for bruises, inflammation or oedema

A. Sub cut: palpate sites for masses or tenderness. Avoid these areas. For daily insulin, rotate site daily. Be sure the needle is correct size by grasping skin fold at site with thumb and forefinger. Measure fold from top to bottom; needle should be half length

B. IM: note integrity, size of muscle, and palpate for tenderness or hardness. Avoid these areas if injections are given frequently, rotate sites

Help patient to comfortable position:

- Sub cut
  - Have patient relax arm, leg or abdomen, depending on site chosen for injection
- IM
  - Have patient lie flat on side or prone, depending on site chosen
- ID
  - Have the patient extend elbow and support it and forearm on a flat surface

  Clean site with an antiseptic swab as appropriate
  Remove needle cap from needle
  Hold syringe between thumb and forefinger of dominant hand:
- Sub cut
  - Hold as dart, palm down or hold syringe across tops of fingertips
- IM
  - Hold as dart, palm down
- ID
  - Hold the bevel of needle pointing up

Administer injection
Subcutaneous
- For average-size patient, spread skin tightly across injection site or pinch skin with non-dominant hand
- Inject needle quickly and firmly at 45- to 90-degree angle. Then release skin, if pinched
- For obese patient, pinch skin at site and inject needle at 90-degree angle below tissue fold
- Inject medication at a steady rate

Intramuscular
- Position non-dominant hand at correct anatomical landmarks
- If patient's muscle mass is small, grasp body of muscle between thumb and fingers
- Insert needle quickly at 90-degree angle
- Inject medication at a steady rate
- Smoothly and steadily withdraw needle and release skin
- Place appropriate dressing over injection site

Intradermal
- With non-dominant hand, stretch skin over site with forefinger or thumb
- With needle against patient's skin, insert it slowly at 5- to 15-degree angle until resistance is felt. Then advance needle through epidermis to approximately 3 mm (about 0.12 inch) below skin surface. Needle tips can be seen through skin
- Inject medication slowly. Normally, resistance is felt. If not, the needle is too deep; remove and begin again

- While injecting medication, notice that a small bleb approximately 6 mm resembling mosquito bite appears on skin's surface

Withdraw needle while applying gauze gently over site. Support of tissue around injection site minimises discomfort during needle withdrawal

Do not massage after sub cut injection of heparin or insulin, or after IM or ID injection

Help patient to comfortable position

Safety needles should be used; when completed, retract needle or click shield over needle to ensure safety. (Warning to paediatric patient of possible 'clicking' noise of needle retraction/shield covering may be required)

Remove disposable gloves and perform hand hygiene

Stay with the patient for 3–5 min and observe for any adverse reactions

Ask whether the patient feels any acute pain, burning, numbness or tingling at injection site

Inspect site, noting any bruising or induration

Return to evaluate patient's response to medication in 10–30 min. IM medications absorb quickly; undesired effects may also develop rapidly

Ask the patient to explain the purpose and effects of medication

For ID injections, use skin pencil and draw circle around perimeter of injection site

Documentation
- Record administration of medication on paediatric NIMIC and add both appropriately qualified nurses' initials, signature or appropriate electronic identifier
- Report any adverse reactions an appropriately qualified nurse or prescriber

(Adapted from Rebeiro et al 2021, Children's Health Queensland Hospital and Health Service 2020 Medication administration – intramuscular injection. Available at: https://www.childrens.health.qld.gov.au/__data/assets/pdf_file/0025/179800/medication-administration-intramuscular-injection.pdf.)

References

AMH Australian Children's Dosing Companion 2022 Average weight and height according to age. Online. Available: https://childrens.amh.net.au/.

Anderson CE, Herring RA 2019 Padiatric Nursing Interventions and Skills. In: MJ Hockenberry, D Wilson, CC Rodgers (eds) Wong's Nursing care of infants and children. Elsevier, St Louis, pp 708–709.

Asthma Australia 2021 About asthma. Asthma is a lifelong condition of the airways. Online. Available: https://asthma.org.au/about-asthma/.

Australian Commission on Safety and Quality in Health Care 2019 National Inpatient Medication Chart (NIMC) – Paediatric. Online. Available: https://www.safetyandquality.gov.au/publications-and-resources/resource-library/national-inpatient-medication-chart-nimc-paediatric.

Australian Commission on Safety and Quality in Health Care 2022 APINCHS classification of high risk medicines. Online. Available: https://www.safetyandquality.gov.au/our-work/medication-safety/high-risk-medicines/apinchs-classification-high-risk-medicines.

Australian Government, Department of Health and Aged Care 2018 Australian immunisation handbook. Online. Available: https://immunisation-handbook.health.gov.au/.

Australian Government, Institute of Health and Welfare 2022 Health literacy. Online. Available: https://www.aihw.gov.au/reports/australias-health/health-literacy. Accessed 1 Aug 2023.

AMH Australian Children's Dosing Companion 2023 Australian Medicines Handbook. Average weight and height according to age. Online. Available: https://childrens.amh.net.au/.

Badaczewski A, Bauman LJ, Blank AE et al 2017 Relationship between teach-back and patient-centered communication in primary care pediatric encounters. Patient Education and Counseling 100 (7): 1345–1352.

Bastable S 2016 Essentials of patient education. Jones & Bartlett Learning, Burlington.

Bryant J, Rance J, Hull P et al 2019 Making sense of 'side effects': counterpublic health in the era of direct-acting antivirals. The International Journal on Drug Policy 72: 77–83.

Children's Health Queensland Hospital and Health Service 2022 Policies and procedures. Peripheral intravenous cannula (PIVC) taping. Online. Available: https://www.childrens.health.qld.gov.au/wp-content/uploads/peripheral-intravenous-cannula-PIVC-taping-nursing-skill-sheet.pdf.

Children's Health Queensland Hospital and Health Service 2020 Medication administration – intramuscular injection. Online. Available: https://www.childrens.health.qld.gov.au/wp-content/uploads/PDF/qpec/nursing-skill-sheets/medication-administration-intramuscular-injection.pdf.

Crisp J, Taylor C, Douglas C, Rebeiro, G 2013 Potter and Perry's Fundamentals of nursing, 4th edn. Elsevier.

Fleming ND, Mills C 1992 Not another inventory, rather a catalyst for reflection. To Improve the Academy 11(1): 137–155.

Hand Hygiene Australia 2023 5 moments for hand hygiene. Online. Available: https://www.hha.org.au/hand-hygiene/5-moments-for-hand-hygiene.

Hockenberry MJ, Wilson D, Rodgers CC 2017 Wong's essentials of pediatric nursing, 10th edn. Elsevier, St Louis.

Hockenberry MJ, Wilson D, Rodgers CC 2019 Wong's nursing care of infants and children, 11th edn. St Louis, Elsevier.

Horeczko T, Enriquez B, McGrath NE et al 2013 The pediatric assessment triangle: accuracy of its application by nurses in the triage of children. Journal of Emergency Nursing 39(2): 182–189.

International Association for the Study of Pain 2023 Revised definition of pain. Online. Available: https://www.iasp-pain.org/publications/iasp-news/iasp-announces-revised-definition-of-pain/.

Jennings P 2024 Paramedic principles and practice in the UK. Elsevier, Oxford.

Kitchie S 2006 Determinants of learning. Essentials of Patient Education, 65–101.

Lilley L, Legge D, Plover C et al 2019 Paediatric injectable guidelines 2019. Royal Children's Hospital – Pharmacy Department. Melbourne, Australia.

Merkel S, Voepel-Lewis T, Shayevitz J et al 1997 The FLACC: a behavioral scale for scoring postoperative pain in young children. Pediatric Nursing 23(3): 293–297.

MIMS Australia 2020 Online. Available: https://app.emims.plus/medicineview?id=815b78d9-ec4b-4d9e-a4b0-a53300fd5ae1&type=abbpi. Accessed 5 Jan 2024.

National Asthma Council Australia 2023 The National Asthma Council Australia. Online. Available: www.nationalasthma.org.au.

Osborne RH, Elmer S, Hawkins M et al 2022 Health literacy development is central to the prevention and control of non-communicable diseases. BMJ Global Health 7: e010362.

Pasero C, McCaffery M 2011 Pain: assessment and pharmacologic management. Mosby, St Louis.

Pfizer Inc. 2023 The newest vital sign. Online. Available: https://www.pfizer.com/products/medicine-safety/health-literacy/nvs-toolkit. Accessed 1 Aug 2023.

Queensland Government, Children's Health 2021 Children's Resuscitation Emergency Drug Dosage (CREDD). Online. Available: https://www.childrens.health.qld.gov.au/for-health-professionals/queensland-paediatric-emergency-care-qpec/emergency-medicine-guides.

Queensland Government, Children's Health Queensland 2022 Asthma – emergency management in children. Online. Available: https://www.childrens.health.qld.gov.au/guideline-asthma-emergency-management-in-children/.

Queensland Government, Children's Health Queensland 2022 Puffers and spacers. Online. Available: https://www.childrens.health.qld.gov.au/fact-sheet-puffers-and-spacers/.

Queensland Government 2023 Queensland Health Mental Health Act 2016 Guide to patient rights. Online. Available: https://www.health.qld.gov.au/__data/assets/pdf_file/0031/444856/guide-to-mha.pdf.

Queensland Health, Clinical Excellence Queensland 2023 Guide to informed decision-making in health care, Interim update, version 2.2. Online. Available: https://www.health.qld.gov.au/__data/assets/pdf_file/0019/143074/ic-guide.pdf. Accessed 4 Jan 2024.

Queensland Government, Queensland Ambulance Service 2022 Clinical practice manual (CPM). Online. Available: https://www.ambulance.qld.gov.au/clinical.html.

Queensland Government 2022 Queensland Legislation. Child Protection Act 1999. Online. Available: https://www.legislation.qld.gov.au.

Queensland Government, Children's Health Queensland 2023 Queensland paediatric emergency care (QPEC). Online. Available: https://www.childrens.health.qld.gov.au/chq/health-professionals/qld-paediatric-emergency-care/.

Ramasamy S, Baysari MT, Lehnbom E et al 2013 Evidence briefings on interventions to improve medication safety: double-checking medication administration. University of New South Wales. Online. Available: https://www.safetyandquality.gov.au/publications/evidence-briefings-on-interventions-to-improve-medication-safety-double-checking-medication-administration/.

Rebeiro G, Wilson D, Fuller S 2021 Fundamentals of nursing: clinical skills workbook, 4th edn. Elsevier, NSW.

Tiziani A 2020 Havard's nursing guide to drugs, 10th edn. Elsevier Australia, Sydney.

The Royal Australian and New Zealand College of Psychiatrists 2023 Mental health legislation Australia and Aotearoa New Zealand. Online. Available: https://www.ranzcp.org/clinical-guidelines-publications/in-focus-topics/mental-health-legislation. Accessed 1 Aug 2023.

The Royal Children's Hospital Melbourne 2001 How to give medications to children. Online. Available: https://www.rch.org.au/uploadedFiles/Main/Content/pharmacy/how-to-give-medications-to-children.pdf.

The Royal Children's Hospital Melbourne 2020 Kids Health Information. CVAD: peripherally inserted central catheter PICC. Online. Available: https://www.rch.org.au/kidsinfo/fact_sheets/CVAD__Peripherally_Inserted_Central_Catheter_PICC/.

The Royal Children's Hospital Melbourne 2020 Kids Health Information. CVAD: port. Online. Available: https://www.rch.org.au/kidsinfo/fact_sheets/CVAD__Port/.

The Royal Children's Hospital Melbourne 2020 Kids Health Information. CVAD: tunnelled – centrally inserted central line T-CICC. Online. Available: https://www.rch.org.au/kidsinfo/fact_sheets/CVAD__Tunnelled_Cuffed_-_Centrally_Inserted_Central_Catheter_TC-CICC/.

The Royal Children's Hospital Melbourne 2022 Clinical Practice Guidelines. Pain assessment and measurement. Online. Available: https://www.rch.org.au/clinicalguide/.

The Royal Children's Hospital Melbourne. Clinical Guidelines (Nursing). Subcutaneous catheter devices management of insuflon and BD saf-T-Intima devices. Online. Available: https://www.rch.org.au/rchcpg/hospital_clinical_guideline_index/Subcutaneous_catheter_devices_management_of_insuflon_and_BD_safTIntima_devices/. Accessed 4 August 2023.

Workman ML, LaCharity LA 2016 Understanding pharmacology: essentials for medication safety, 2nd edn. Elsevier.

World Health Organization (WHO) 2019 5 moments for medication safety. Online. Available: https://www.who.int/publications/i/item/WHO-HIS-SDS-2019.4.

Further reading

Queensland Government 2022 Queensland Health. Infection prevention and control guidance (including PPE advice). Online. Available: https://www.health.qld.gov.au/clinical-practice/guidelines-procedures/novel-coronavirus-qld-clinicians/personal-protective-equipment-ppe.

Queensland Government 2023 Queensland Legislation. Online. Available: https://www.legislation.qld.gov.au.

Queensland Health 2022 Patient Safety and Quality. Recognising and Responding to Acute Deterioration (RRAD). Online. Available: https://qheps.health.qld.gov.au/psu/rrad/rrad-ewars-forms.

Queensland Health 2023 Personal Protective Equipment. Online. Available: https://www.health.qld.gov.au/clinical-practice/guidelines-procedures/novel-coronavirus-qld-clinicians/personal-protective-equipment/ppe.

The Royal Australian and New Zealand College of Psychiatrists 2017 Mental health legislation Australia and Aotearoa New Zealand. Informed consent – mental health legislation. Online. Available: https://www.ranzcp.org/clinical-guidelines-publications/in-focus/topics/mental-health-legislation.

Westbrook JI, Li L, Lehnbom EC et al 2015 What are incident reports telling us? A comparative study at two Australian hospitals of medication errors identified at audit, detected by staff and reported to an incident system. International Journal for Quality in Health Care: Journal of the International Society for Quality in Health Care 27(1): 1–9.

Useful websites/ information

CONTACT AND DROPLET PRECAUTIONS. YouTube – https://www.youtube.com/watch?v=JKBfRHG5X90

Diabetes Australia – https://www.diabetesaustralia.com.au/

Drop the jargon – https://www.youtube.com/watch?v=M7KmxTgLZ6k

Website from Government of Western Australia. South Metropolitan Health Service

Drop the jargon – Health Literacy Video – https://pipsmhs.health.wa.gov.au/drop-jargon

How a tunnelled central line is placed. YouTube – https://www.youtube.com/watch?v=nhCuebdcTEI

Pate JW, Noblet T, Hush JM et. al 2019 Exploring the concept of pain of Australian children with and without pain: qualitative study. BMJ Open 2019; 9(10): e033199

An article of interest to assist the paediatric nurse with the assessment of pain

Physical Hold vs Restraint or Seclusion. Behavioral Health. Care Treatment and Services CTS. The Joint Commission – http://tinyurl.com/3y2wt8ar

Preisz A, Preisz P 2019 Restraint in paediatrics: a delicate balance. Journal of Paediatrics and Child Health 55(10): 1165–1169

The above journal article provides insight into this delicate topic

This is bad enough: a poem by Elspeth Murray – https://www.youtube.com/watch?v=R3tJ-MXqPmk

TLC for Kids' Distraction Box Program – https://www.tlcforkids.org.au/distraction-box-program/

https://www.rch.org.au/uploadedFiles/Main/Content/ethics/Writing%20Tips.pdf

This resource from the Royal Children's Hospital Melbourne has useful information for using plain language

Index

155